A Course in Clinical Disorders
of the Body Fluids and
Electrolytes

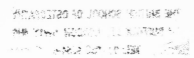

In memory of my father
Charles S. Berlyne
1892 – 1979

A Course in Clinical Disorders of the Body Fluids and Electrolytes

GEOFFREY M. BERLYNE

MD, FRCP, FACP
Professor of Medicine
Downstate Medical Center
State University of New York;
Co-Director,
Division of Renal Diseases
Downstate Medical Center,
Brooklyn,
Chief, Section of Nephrology,
Brooklyn V A Medical Center,
Brooklyn, New York

BLACKWELL SCIENTIFIC PUBLICATIONS

OXFORD   LONDON   EDINBURGH   BOSTON   MELBOURNE

© 1980 by Blackwell Scientific Publications
Editorial offices:
Osney Mead, Oxford, OX2 OEL
8 John Street, London, WC1N 2ES
9 Forrest Road, Edinburgh, EH1 2QH
52 Beacon Street, Boston, Mass., USA
214 Berkeley Street, Carlton
Victoria 3053, Australia

First published 1980

DISTRIBUTORS

USA
Blackwell Mosby Book Distributors
11830 Westline Industrial Drive
St Louis, Missouri 63141

Canada
Blackwell Mosby Book Distributors
86 Northline Road, Toronto
Ontario, M4B 3E5

Australia
Blackwell Scientific Book
Distributors
214 Berkeley Street, Carlton
Victoria 3053

British Library
Cataloguing in Publication Data
Berlyne, Geoffrey Merton
A course in clinical disorders of
the body fluids and electrolytes.
1. Water-electrolyte imbalances —
Programmed instructions
I. Title
616.3′9   RC630
ISBN 0-632-00356-1

Photoset, printed and bound in Malta by Interprint Limited

Contents

This book is dedicated to Eli A. Friedman M.D.,
a good and wise colleague, and
an accomplished nephrophile.

Introduction

This book is aimed at the senior medical student, the MRCP candidate and hospital resident who frequently has difficulty in understanding the principles of management of fluid and electrolyte problems. Having spent many years in correcting fluid and electrolyte imbalances with resident hospital staff in various countries, I thought that a semi-programmed course on disorders of the body fluids and electrolytes was necessary. I have put it in a semi-programmed form like its companion volume, *A Course in Renal Diseases*, so that the reader cannot day-dream while reading the book. I believe that the intelligent reader will grasp the essentials of fluid and electrolyte problems from this book more readily than from standard form texts and so will be better able to appreciate the more detailed review articles on the subjects should he wish to have a deeper knowledge.

This book is printed in a small, soft-back format to enable the reader to keep it in his coat pocket, and read it whenever he has a chance. The times for each chapter are but a rough guide. Most chapters are too long to be completed at one sitting; and no one should read for more than 30 minutes at one time.

The programming instructions must be followed. This means that the paragraphs are deliberately scrambled to prevent anyone from browsing through the book. I hope the reader enjoys using the book as a pocket teaching machine.

For those readers living in countries where SI units are used, I have printed the SI values in italics, but have kept the standard (mass) units in regular print.

I would like to thank my colleagues, and the residents, fellows, and students of our renal programme at Downstate Medical Center, State University of New York, for reading the chapters as they were prepared and making appropriate and valuable suggestions to improve the text. Dr. E. Goldberger gave kind permission to reproduce several of the figures from his book, *A Primer of Electrolyte and Acid—Base Disorders*, 5th Edition. Lea & Febiger.

New York, March 1979   **G. M. Berlyne**

How to Use This Book

In each chapter:

1 Follow the programme instructions.
2 Stop for at least 15 minutes after every 30 minutes' learning. This makes your learning more efficient and your life more bearable.
3 Never use the index until you have read the entire book.
4 Follow the printed order of the chapters.

Time for this chapter: $1\frac{1}{2}$ hours

Chapter 1
Body fluids

1.1 Water is the principal constituent by weight of the mammalian body. The various tissues have different water contents, thus the water content of the brain is 82 per cent by weight, whereas the water content of bone is 20 per cent by weight. The lowest water content is found in adipose tissue which has a water content of 10 per cent. Look at Table 1.1 in which the water content of the various tissues is compared.

Table 1.1

Tissue	Water content as %
Brain	82
Skeletal muscle	76
Liver	68
Kidney	83
Blood	83
Skin	72
Bone	22
Adipose tissue	10

In the average man there is less fat than in the average woman, so that the percentage of water in the average male body will be higher than in the female body. This is shown below:

Sex	Water content as % of total body weight
Male	60.6
Female	50.2

Now answer the question:

Question What tissue has the lowest water content?

1

Answer 1. Bone. Go on to **1.3**.
2. Fat. Go on to **1.4**.
3. Muscle. Go on to **1.6**.

1.2 You should not be reading this. Read **1.1** again and follow the instructions, otherwise you are wasting your time.

1.3 Your answer— bone.

You are not correct. Bone has 22 per cent water content whereas fat has only 10 per cent. Look again at Table 1.1 and answer the question correctly.

1.4 Your answer—fat has the lowest water content.

You are correct.

Obviously a fat man will have a lower percentage of water in his body than will be found in a thin woman. If an average man weighs 70 kg and of this 60 per cent is water, then the absolute amount of water in his body will be $70 \times 60/100 = 42$ litres. This quantity of water is referred to as Total Body Water or TBW. Total Body Water can be measured by several methods:

1. Desiccation. This method is suitable for small animals and consists of weighing the animal before and after drying the carcass to constant weight in an oven for a few days at 95°C. This is not suitable for large animals or man for obvious reasons, but is a method which is free of major error for small laboratory animals.

2. Dilution methods. The principle of these methods is the administration of a known quantity of a substance which readily diffuses throughout the water in the entire body. After equilibrium has been attained (which may take several hours), the concentration of the administered substance is determined in the plasma and from this observed dilution of the substance, the volume of its distribution determined, with an appropriate correction for the loss of the substance excreted from the body. If a marker is used which distributes throughout body water then this volume of distribution is Total Body Water.

TBW = Volume of distribution.
$$= \frac{\text{Quantity administered— Quantity excreted.}}{\text{Concentration of marker in plasma water.}}$$

Question If you have to determine Total Body Water repeatedly in the same man, what type of method would you use?
Answer 1. Desiccation. Go on to **1.5**.
          2. Dilution. Go on to **1.7**.
          3. Don't know. Go on to **1.8**.

1.5 Your answer—desiccation.
You are wrong. Can you place a man in an oven at 95°C and dry him out and then expect him to live and repeat the experiment? You are not thinking, try and concentrate. Read **1.4** again.

1.6 Your answer— muscle.
You are guessing. You must concentrate on what you are reading. Go back and re-read **1.1** and pay particular attention to the Table.

1.7 Your answer— dilution methods should be used to measure Total Body Water in man.
You are correct. The substances which can be used for the measurements of total body water should have the following properties—

1. Diffuse throughout the body water.
2. Should not be specifically bound to any cellular or extracellular component.
3. Metabolized either not at all or very slowly.
4. Readily measured accurately.
5. Non-toxic.

Commonly used substances are:
(1) Antipyrene, a chemical compound introduced initially in the treatment of pyrexia, and easily measured chemically. It is slowly excreted and slowly metabolized.
(2) Isotopes of water,—deuterium hydroxide (D_2O) and tritiated water (^3H_2O) are treated by the body as if they were ordinary water, and are particularly suitable for the determination of total body water. Deuterium oxide is expensive and for its accurate measurement a mass spectrograph is required which is costly and not available in every hospital. Tritiated water, on the other hand, is not expensive and is readily measured in a liquid scintillation counter usually to be found in nuclear medicine laboratories of all major hospitals. These measurements using isotopes of water give Total Body Water results which are identical.

They are however, about 2 litres greater than the result of the antipyrene determined total body water volume, presumably due to deuterium and tritium exchanging with isotopic hydrogen in proteins and carbohydrates.

(3) In experimental animals, urea, alcohol, and thiosulphate are substances used to measure total body water, but urea and alcohol are both metabolized and about 10 g or more of urea is also concomitantly produced in the body during the time of equilibration. This makes them less ideal than tritiated water for measuring Total Body Water.

Question If you do repeated total body water measurements on the same subject would you expect the results from antipyrene or thiosulphate to be identical with those obtained by using tritiated water?

Answer 1. Yes. Go on to **1.9**.
2. No. Go on to **1.10**.

1.8 Your answer— I don't know.

How could you choose this? You should have read **1.4** again if you were unable to choose the correct answer. An answer such as 'I don't know' is an admission of ignorance of the contents of **1.4**. Go back and re-read it. Then choose the correct answer without guesswork. Don't waste your time.

1.9 Your answer— yes.

TBW is the same by both methods. No. You have not read **1.7** carefully enough. Tritiated water gives a larger TBW space than is found with antipyrene or thiosulphate methods read **1.7** again to find out why.

1.10 Your answer— different results of Total Body Water are obtained depending on the method used.

You are correct. From Paragraph **1.7** there is a simple lesson to be learned:

That using the usual chemical or physical methods of measurement of Total Body Water gives results which may vary due to the method used, and *it is, therefore, extremely important to define the method used when describing Total Body Water*. Changes in Total Body Water (TBW) are not meaningful if, for example, before the experimental stress TBW is measured say by tritiated water, and after the stress by antipyrene. The methods usually employed are sufficiently reproducible to be dependable and sensitive enough to show small changes if the same test is repeated. In clinical practice, however, the easiest and most accurate test of a change in total body water over a period of a few hours or days is by measuring the *change in body weight* determined by weighing the patient. Apart from actual removal of tissue or fluid in surgical operations and childbirth, a rapid change in body weight is a good indication of a change in total body water.

In the pregnant woman there is an increase in total body water as measured by deuterium of about 7 litres after the end of the first trimester, not accompanied by clinical oedema. About half of this is attributable to the water content of the pregnant uterus, fetus and amniotic fluid.

In the neonate, infant and child the total body water as expressed as a percentage of body weight differs from that in the adults. Look at Table 1.10.

The relatively high body water content of the infant and child, compared to adult man is due to the higher percentage of extracellular fluid in the infant and child compared to the intracellular fluid.

Question There is an increased amount of TBW per kg of body weight in the infant compared with the adult. What is the reason for this?:

Answer 1. Increase in percentage of ECF. Go on to **1.12**.
2. Increase in relative amounts of both ECF and ICF. Go on to **1.14**.
3. Increase in relative amount of internal organs compared to whole body weight. Go on to **1.16**.

Table 1.10

Age	Total body water (%)	Ratio of extracellular fluid to intracellular fluid
0–1 days	79	1.25
1–10 days	74	1.14
1–3 months	72.3	0.80
3–6 months	70.1	0.75
6–12 months	60.4	0.83
2–3 years	63.5	0.73
5–10 years	61.5	0.56
10–16 years	58	0.48

1.11 Your answer— The ECF provides the milieu interieur.
You are correct.

ECF is divided into 4 compartments:

1. Intravascular fluid compartment.
2. Extravascular fluid compartment.
3. Inaccessible bone water.
4. Transcellular fluids.

Let us consider each of them in turn—

First of all, the intravascular compartment. This is the plasma inside the vascular tree i.e. inside the heart chambers, the arteries and veins of all sizes, and the capillaries. It excludes the cellular components of the blood— the red cells, white cells and platelets, which are part of the intracellular compartment. The plasma is in equilibrium with the extravascular part of the ECF. The plasma is unique in its high protein concentration of 6 to 7 g/100 ml, which is important in maintaining an adequate oncotic pressure in the capillaries and attracting interstitial fluid back into the intravascular compartment. Oncotic pressure is the osmotic pressure exerted by colloids i.e. large molecules. In healthy man, the plasma proteins are the main factor contributing to oncotic pressure. The capillaries are permeable to small molecules, but not to large molecules, thus the osmotic pressure exerted by small molecules such as electrolytes is unimportant in the capillaries where larger molecules, such as colloids, exert oncotic pressure which attracts fluid back into the capillaries.

Read this last paragraph again after you have looked at the diagram. Draw the diagram yourself. See how the plasma proteins exert oncotic pressure and pull the fluid *back* into the capillary: hydrostatic pressure does the opposite. The result is an equilibrium.

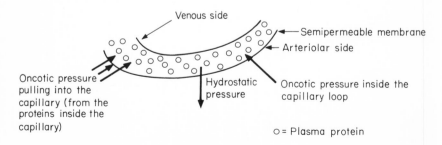

Fig. 1.11

Now answer the question.

Question What is plasma oncotic pressure?

Answer 1. Osmotic pressure of electrolytes. Go on to **1.17**.
2. Osmotic pressure of large molecules such as proteins. Go on to **1.19**.

1.12 Your answer— There is an increase in the percentage of ECF in infancy.

You are correct. Total Body Water can be divided into 2 major compartments as you can see in the Fig. 1.12. Look at it carefully, and draw it on a piece of paper. Memorize the figures given for an adult man.

(1) Extracellular fluid compartment (ECF).
(2) Intracellular fluid compartment (ICF).

The concept of compartments is perhaps not really adequate. A better description is that of Robinson and McCance (1952) who likened the ECF to the continuous phase of an emulsion and the ICF to the disperse phase. A more appropriate description would be to liken the body fluid to a solution in which micelles were suspended. The ECF is then the continuous phase and the ICF analogous to the fluid contents of the micelles themselves.

The ECF is an all-pervading fluid surrounding the cells. It is kept constant in composition within fairly narrow limits, so that it is, in truth, the constant 'milieu interieur' or internal milieu of Claude Bernard, in which osmolality, chemical and ionic composition and pH are rigidly controlled. Thus extremes of diet i.e. (from starvation to gluttony) over- and under-hydration, and activity have minimal effects on the composition of the EFC and the cells are thereby protected from changes in their external environment.

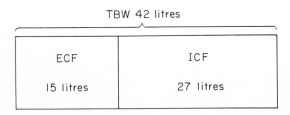

Fig. 1.12   Relative sizes of extracellular and intracellular compartments.

Question What provides the constant milieu interieur?

Answer 1. The ECF. Go on to **1.11**.
2. The ICF. Go on to **1.13**.
3. Total Body Water. Go on to **1.15**.

1.13 Your answer— the ICF provides the milieu interieur.

No. The continuous phase of the body fluids is the ECF, which provides the milieu interieur. The ICF composition varies from cell to cell, there being differences in, for instance, the pH in the muscle cell when compared to pH in the leucocyte, as well as differences *inside* the cell in the various subcellular compartments i.e. mitochondria, lysosomes, cytosol, endoplasmic reticulum, and nuclei. Constancy of the milieu interieur is a function of the ECF, not the ICF. Read **1.12** again. It is best to consider the cystol as the ICF and the subcellular particles as each having their own pH, ionic composition and metabolic functions i.e. islands in the cytosol.

1.14 Your answer— There is an increase in the relative amounts of both ECF and ICF.

You are partially correct, but you have not based your answer on **1.10**. Go back and read it, paying particular attention to the Table. Then answer the question correctly.

1.15 Your answer— Total body water provides the milieu interieur.

No. You have not read **1.12** properly. Re-read it. There is no point in guessing. If you cannot concentrate stop reading now and begin again when you can devote your attention to the writing without distraction.

1.16 Your answer— There is an increase in the relative amount of internal organs.

You are correct, but this is not the reason stated in **1.10**. Read **1.10** again and you will find that there is an increase in the amount of ECF kg body weight in childhood when compared with that in adults.

1.17 Your answer— Oncotic pressure is the osmotic pressure of electrolytes.

No. This is not so. It is the osmotic pressure of the large molecules such as proteins. Read **1.11** again more carefully.

Table 1.18

Electrolytes		ECF Interstitial plasma fluid	Interstitial fluid	ICF
Cations mEq/l	Na^+	142	145	10
	K^+	4	4	155
	$Ca_2{}^+$	5	—	3
	$Mg_2{}^+$	2	—	26
Total		153		194
Anions mEq/l	Cl^-	104	114	2
	HCO_3^-	27	31	8
	HPO_4^{2-}	2	—	95
	SO_4^{2-}	1	—	20
	Organic acids	6	—	
	Protein	13		15
Total		153		180

1.18   Your answer— The deeper layers of bone.

You are correct. The composition of extracellular fluid is shown in Table 1.18. Plasma differs from extravascular or interstitial fluid in that the latter has a lower protein content, and there are minor differences in electrolyte composition caused by the Gibbs—Donnan distribution factor. This is discussed later. Meanwhile remember that the **principal cation in ECF is sodium** i.e. it has the highest concentration and sodium is **therefore osmotically the most important of the cations**, with chloride and bicarbonate being the major anions in ECF. All other ions are in lower concentration. This is in striking contrast to the composition of intracellular fluid (ICF) which has high concentrations of potassium, magnesium, phosphate, sulphate and protein. ICF is discussed in detail later.

Now answer the question:

Question   What is the osmotically most important cation of the ECF?

Answer   1. Potassium. Go on to **1.21**.
          2. Sodium. Go on to **1.23**.

1.19   Your answer—oncotic pressure is osmotic pressure exerted by large molecules such as proteins.

You are correct. The extravascular or interstitial fluid is the fluid

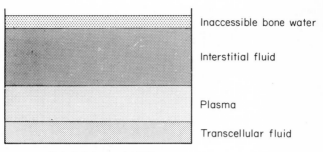

Subdivisions of ECF

Fig. 1.19

surrounding the cells, and is in equilibrium with the intravascular plasma and with the fluid inside the cells (ICF). The interstitial fluid includes lymph, and mostly achieves rapid equilibrium with the plasma. However, in contrast to this the interstitial fluid of cartilage and dense connective tissue is in slow equilibrium with plasma, due to the physical gel-like structure of the intercellular tissue.

Transcellular fluids are the secretions of glandular tissues such as saliva, gastro-intestinal fluids, renal tract, respiratory tract, gonads, aqueous humour, and the cerebrospinal fluid. Inaccessible Bone Water is the water which is trapped in the deep layers of bone and is not readily exchangeable with the remainder of the ECF.

Now answer the question.

Question Where is the inaccessible bone water?

Answer 1. In the superficial layers of bone. Go on to **1.20**.
2. In the deeper layers of bone. Go on to **1.18**.

1.20 Your answer— inaccessible bone water is in the superficial layers of bone.

You are wrong. Inaccessible bone water is in the deeper layers of bone. Being surrounded by bone makes it not readily exchangeable and out of contact with the remaining ECF. Read **1.19**.

1.21 Your answer— potassium is the most osmotically active cation in the ECF.

You are not correct. Potassium is found in low concentrations in ECF (around 4 mM/1) whereas plasma sodium concentration, you will remember, is of the order of 140 mM/1. Now read **1.18** again and answer the question correctly.

1.22   Your answer— blood volume is 40 ml/kg. You are correct.

Total ECF volume can be measured by substances which diffuse through the ECF but do not penetrate the cells. At the outset it should be realized that no such ideal substance exists. Measurements of ECF volume by large molecule polysaccharides (such as in inulin) are far from satisfactory because they fail to penetrate all the ECF, as shown by the fact that the inulin space of guinea pig muscle increases after administration of hyaluronidase, suggesting an extracellular mucopolysaccharide barrier to the diffusion of inulin. On the other hand, bromide and chloride apparently penetrate into some cells, and so give values of ECF much higher than inulin space. Look at Table 1.22.

Sulphate labelled with ^{35}S gives a modest ECF space estimate suggesting failure to penetrate readily into cells. When $^{35}SO_4^{2-}$ and inulin spaces are compared for the various tissues, $^{35}SO_4^{2-}$ penetrates transcellular spaces which inulin does not penetrate. It is important to realize that there is no substance which measures ECF space absolutely; each method measures a different space. The changes in that particular space in a variety of circumstances can be accurately measured by repeating the test with the **same** tracer (or the same chemical).

Now answer the question.

Question Which gives the lowest value for ECF space?

Answer   1. Bromide. Go on to **1.29**.
             2. Inulin. Go on to **1.27**.
             3. Sulphate. Go on to **1.30**.

Table 1.22

Method	ECF space (expressed as % body weight)
Inulin	16
Thiosulphate	16
$^{35}SO_4^{2-}$	18
$^{86}Br^-$	28
$^{36}Cl^-$	27

1.23   Your answer— sodium is the most osmotically active cation of the ECF.

You are correct. Sodium is the cation responsible for the maintenance of ECF volume as a constant, and much of the kidneys' oxygen consumption is devoted to tubular absorption of sodium to maintain a normal ECF volume.

Measurement of ECF volume can be divided into: (1) measurement of plasma volume (which is in day to day use in assessing fluid requirements, in patients with fluid and electrolyte balance disturbances). (2) Measurements of total ECF volume (which is primarily a research procedure).

Plasma volume. Plasma volume can be measured by direct dilution methods involving the dilution of a protein bound dye such as Evan's Blue (T1824), or radioactive human serum albumin (RISA) labelled with ^{125}I. Indirect methods are available which involve measuring red cell mass by labelling red cells with ^{51}Cr and then determining plasma volume from the whole body haematocrit.

An example of this is worth working through because you will very likely need to do the test clinically sooner or later in patients suffering from blood loss or fluid and electrolyte disturbances.

^{125}**IHSA test.** 5—10 μC of ^{125}IHSA (Radio-iodinated human serum albumin) are given from a calibrated syringe. An identical dose is made up into a 1/1000 dilution in a solution containing 1g of albumin in 0.9 per cent NaCl. After 10 minutes a heparinized blood sample is taken from a vein in the opposite arm. Aliquots of the standard, plasma and whole blood are counted in a scintillation well type γ counter.

Plasma volume =

$$\frac{\text{counts/min/ml of standard} \times \text{dilution of standard} \times \text{vol of IHSA}}{\text{counts/min/ml of post-injection plasma}}$$

$$\text{Plasma volume} = \frac{\text{Administered dose in cpm}}{\text{cpm per ml of plasma}}$$

The administered dose is calculated from the radioactivity of the standard minus the radioactivity remaining in the syringe.

Let us work through an example. 1 ml of ^{125}IHSA (approximately 5 μC) were given.

1 ml of 1/1000 dilution of standard solution has 14,000 cpm/ml

∴ Administered dose = 14,000,000 cpm

1 ml of plasma taken after 20 min has 5000 cpm/ml.

$$\text{Plasma volume} = \frac{\text{administered dose in cpm}}{\text{cpm/ml of plasma}} = \frac{14,000,000}{5,000}$$

$$= 2,800 \text{ ml.}$$

If weight of patient is 70 kg,

then Plasma volume = 2800/70 ml/kg = *40 ml/kg*.

Injection of Evans' Blue (T1824) is a useful non-radioactive dilution method of measuring plasma volume. An injection of a known quantity of the dye is given and plasma volume determined from a sample of blood taken at 5, 10, 15 and 20 minutes. The dye is bound to protein in the plasma. The concentration in standard solutions and plasma is measured in a colorimeter, the calculation being made after a standard curve of dye concentration versus optical density has been made, the colorimeter readings being converted to mg of dye/ml, and extrapolation made for the concentration of dye at the time of injection.

$$\text{Plasma volume} = \frac{\text{mg of T1824 administered}}{\text{mg of T1824 per ml of plasma}}$$

Neither of these methods is reliable if protein loss occurs from the vascular compartment into other sites (i.e. loss via the kidneys in nephrotic syndrome or loss into ascitic fluid), but this may be negligible in the short time needed for equilibrium. In these circumstances correction has to be made for dye lost into these sites.

Question Below are given the figures from a plasma volume experiment using radioactive ^{125}I labelled HSA. Dose given = 25,000,000 cpm. Plasma radioactivity = 7,500 cpm/ml. Body weight = 83.3 kg. Work out plasma volume in ml per kg body weight.

Answer 1. 45 ml/kg. Go on to **1.24**.
2. 40 ml/kg. Go on to **1.22**.
3. 3333 ml. Go on to **1.25**.

1.24   Your answer— blood volume 45 ml/kg.

You are wrong. The dose given is divided by the counts per ml of plasma. This gives the blood volume for the whole body weight. To obtain blood volume per kg one has to divide the result by the body weight in kg. You have not read **1.23** properly. Now read it again.

1.25   Your answer—blood volume is 3333 ml. You have forgotten to divide by body weight. Go on to **1.23**.

1.26   Your answer—sodium concentration is higher in glomerular filtrate. You have not read **1.27**. Go over it again and choose the correct answer.

1.27   Your answer— inulin gives the lowest value for ECF.

Correct. The Gibbs—Donnan rule states that at equilibrium conditions the product of the concentrations of any pair of diffusable cations and anions on one side of the membrane will be equal to the product of those on the other side. Protein at the pH of plasma (pH 7.4) behaves as an anion. Total anions and total cations must equal each other on each side of the membrane, but because of the large protein 'anionic' molecule there will be fewer non-protein anions and more cations on the side of the membrane where the protein is. Let us look at this in more detail. Look at the situation in Fig. 1.27a which is the status before equilibrium develops. On one side of the semi-permeable membrane there is a protein solution, on the other sodium chloride.

Then the situation is such that both chloride and sodium pass across the membrane into the protein solution, so that at equilibrium, the situation is as shown below in Fig. 1.27b. Because the total anions and total cations are equal *inside* each compartment separately, then the total ions in each of the compartments are shown here. Thus in the protein free compartment, sodium concentration is lower and chloride is higher than

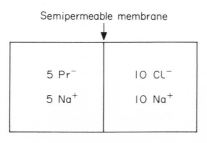

Fig. 1.27a

5 Pr⁻
5 Na⁺
4 Cl⁻
4 Na⁺
6 Cl⁻
6 Na⁺

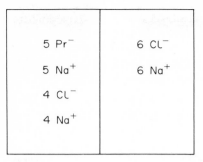

Fig. 1.27b

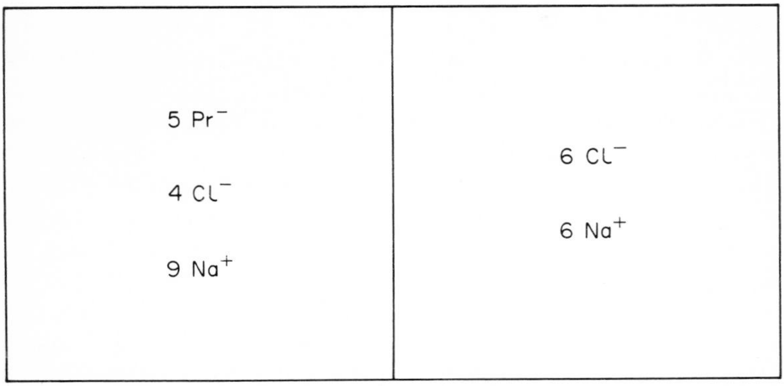

5 Pr⁻
4 Cl⁻
9 Na⁺
6 Cl⁻
6 Na⁺

Fig. 1.27c

in the protein compartment Fig. 1.27c. The ratios between the two compartments for various ions are known as the Gibbs–Donnan factor for that ion.

The concentrations of ions in the plasma should be expressed as mEq per *litre* of plasma *water* because the ions are not dissolved in the 60 or 70g of protein present in plasma. Only then can we compare the concentrations of ions in the plasma with the concentrations in the interstitial fluid.

In practice it has been found that in the interstitial fluid, where there is a relatively low protein content, the concentration of anions is 1.05 times higher than in plasma; the cations are in a concentration of 0.95 times the plasma concentration. This factor of 0.95 or 1.05 depending on whether cations or anions are discussed, is known as the Gibbs—Donnan Factor. It is used in all calculations in which cation and anion concentrations are calculated in plasma ultrafiltrates, whether in the kidney or the interstitial fluid. Read this paragraph again.

Now answer the question.

Question In the glomerular filtrate inside Bowman's space, is the sodium concentration lower than in the plasma or higher?

Answer 1. Lower. Go on to **1.31**.
2. Higher. Go on to **1.26**.

1.28 Your answer— potassium concentration is lower in ICF than in ECF. You have not read **1.30** with adequate concentration.

1.29 Your answer—the lowest value for ECF space is obtained by bromide.

You are wrong. You have not been concentrating. Read **1.22** again.

1.30 Your answer— the lowest value for ECF space is obtained by sulphate. You are not concentrating. Read **1.22** again.

1.31 Your answer— sodium concentration is lower in glomerular filtrate.

You are correct. ICF space is not measured directly, but is calculated as the difference between total body water and extracellular space

$$ICF = TBW - ECF.$$

Measurement of ICF volume, therefore suffers doubly from the inaccuracies inherent in measurement of both TBW and ECF.

The composition of ICF is shown in the Table 1.31 where it is compared to ECF composition. It is a conceptual error to think of the intracellular fluid as an homogeneous entity, with a pH, osmolality and ionic composition which is as uniform as the corresponding factors in the ECF. The ICF consists of a multicompartmental entity, each part of which has its own characteristics depending on its structure and its functional state. Thus it would be an error to expect the pH of the metabolically active mitochondria to have necessarily the same calcium concentration as the cytosol, and indeed with respect to ionized calcium they certainly have different concentrations. Similarly lysosomes, pinocytic vacuoles and the Golgi apparatus all have particular metabolic functions

Table 1.31 Electrolyte composition of the body fluids

Electrolytes	Serum (mEq/litre)	Serum water (mEq/litre)*	Interstitial fluid mEq/litre†	Intracellular fluid (muscle) (mEq/kg H_2O)
Cations:				
Sodium (Na^+)	142	152.7	145	±10
Potassium (K^+)	4	4.3	4	156
Calcium (Ca^{2+})	5	5.4		3.3
Magnesium (Mg^+)	2	2.2		195
Total Cations	153	165	149	195
Anions:				
Chloride (Cl^-)	104	108.5	114	±2
Bicarbonate (HCO)	27	29.3	31	±8
Phosphate (HPO)	2	2.2		95
Sulphate (SO_4^{2-})	1	1		20
Organic acids	6	6.4		
Protein	13	17.2		55
Total Anions:	153	165	145	180+

* Approximate totals only.
† Ignoring all but Na, K, Cl, HCO_3. After R. M. Hays.

and it would be unwise to expect them to be uniform in ionic composition, protein content, enzyme content and pH. Furthermore, from one cell type to another these factors would be as different as they appear to be under the electron microscope. With the best micropuncture methods we get a crude mixture of cytosol and whatever happens to be in it, so that even measurements of ICF potassium ion activity, which are one third of the total cellular potassium in value, are of limited value in understanding what is going on in the various subcellular compartments. Thus the value of whole body intracellular pH or even tissue pH determined by DMO (5,5 dimethyl 2,4 oxazolidonedione) is of dubious relevance to what is going on in a specific subcellular compartment which may be carrying out a vital and characteristic function for that cell, e.g., secretion of a hormone. We have a better chance of knowing what is going on in the elemental composition of the cellular components by use of X ray or electron microprobe analysis which identifies and quantifies the various elements in electron microscope sections of cells, but even this is beset with serious technological problems. The meaning of ICF osmolality is *cytosol* osmolality.

The entire concept of equality between the intracellular osmolality and the ECF osmolality is based on precious little evidence. Look at the table comparing ECF and ICF. You will see that if we look at cations alone the ICF has 195 mEq per litre and the ECF has 149 mEq per litre. Now we must bear in mind that the ICF is not only not homogeneous, but that the osmolality of the ICF is not obtainable by multiplying the cation content by 2, as is the case in the ECF. Why is it not the same? The answer appears to lie in the binding of potassium and magnesium to enzymes and proteins inside the cell, so that they no longer function as osmotically active individual particles. Thus if we measure potassium ion in the cell it is much less than the potassium atomic content as measured with the flame photometer. Similarly we know that only a fraction of magnesium in the cell is exchangeable, and probably the rest is bound so that it cannot contribute to the osmolality of the intracellular fluid, or to be more precise, of the cytosol.

You should read the last paragraph again because it contains some truths which may well have troubled you but which are not much stressed in standard texts on fluid and electrolytes, which treat the ICF as an homogeneous entity.

Question Is the potassium content of ICF higher or lower than in Interstitial fluid of ECF?

Answer 1. Potassium concentration is lower in ICF. Go on to **1.28**.
       2. Potassium concentration is higher in ICF. Go on to **1.32**.
       3. Potassium concentration is equal in ECF and ICF. Go on to **1.33**.

1.32 Your answer—potassium concentration is higher in the ICF.
You are correct. It is worthwhile considering what will happen if we add water or sodium chloride to the ECF. Firstly, let us assume that we drink 3 litres of water rapidly in 20 minutes. Let us also call cytosol osmolality ICF osmolality. The water will first of all be absorbed from the gastro-intestinal tract into the ECF and so expand it to 18 litres (from 15 litres) with a resultant fall in osmolality to $280 \times \frac{15}{18} = 233$ mOsm/kg. There is thus a lower osmolality in the ECF than in cytosol so that then water will enter the ICF from the ECF until the osmolalities of ICF and ECF are equalized again when the ECF will have $\frac{15}{42} \times 3$ litres of extra water, and the ICF $\frac{27}{42} \times 3$ litres of extra water. Of course there is a reduction in ECF osmolality, ADH secretion will cease and a water diuresis will occur until the plasma osmolality has returned to normal i.e., after a diuresis of 3 litres of water. Thus finally, normal ICF and ECF volumes and osmolalities will be restored.
Now answer the question:

Question When water is drunk, into which compartments of the body fluids does it penetrate?

Answer 1. ICF only. Go on to **1.34**.
       2. ECF only. Go on to **1.36**.
       3. Both ICF and ECF. Go on to **1.38**.

1.33 Your answer—potassium concentration is equal in ECF and ICF.
You are wrong. Potassium concentration is much higher in ICF. You need to read **1.30** again. Then answer the question correctly.

1.34 Your answer—it penetrates into the ICF.
You are only partly correct. Water penetrates both compartments ECF and ICF. Read **1.32** again carefully before choosing the correct answer.

1.35 Your answer—sodium chloride causes expansion of the ECF.
You are correct. Expansion of the ECF may be caused by pure salt ingestion alone or by addition of salt and water to the body orally or

intravenously. In the latter case the osmolality of the ECF will be virtually unaltered, but ECF volume will be expanded. The healthy kidney responds with a sodium diuresis; this is partly due to an increase in filtered sodium and partly due to the effect of a decrease in sodium reabsorption caused by a fall in plasma aldosterone levels, and possibly due to a natriuretic hormone about whose existence and identity there is still some dispute.

Expansion of ECF causes the following changes:

1. An increase in body weight.
2. Increase in central venous pressure.
3. Increase in arterial blood pressure.
4. Increase in renal blood flow and glomerular filtration rate.
5. The development of peripheral oedema i.e. oedema of the dependent parts.

The mechanism of this development of *overloading of the circulation* is due to the increase in the intravascular ECF volume i.e. the plasma volume which occurs pari passu with an increase in the interstitial or extravascular part of the ECF. Massive increase in plasma volume may lead to congestive heart failure, particularly in the elderly or the patient with cardiac disease.

Now answer the question.

Question In salt and water loading, congestive heart failure is associated with:

Answer 1. Expansion of ICF volume. Go on to **1.40**.
2. Expansion of ECF volume. Go on to **1.41**.
3. Reduction of ECF volume. Go on to **1.43**.

1.36 Your answer—it penetrates ECF only.

You are partly correct. Read **1.32** again carefully before choosing the correct answer.

1.37 Your answer—sodium chloride causes expansion of ICF.

You are incorrect. Sodium entering the cells is pumped out at once. Read **1.38**.

1.38 Your answer—it penetrates both ICF and ECF.

Correct. If 600 mEq of sodium chloride are imbibed in the form of NaCl tablets then a total of 1200 mOsm are added first of all to the ECF.

This is spread over 15 litres of ECF so that there is an *increase* in ECF osmolality of 1200/15 mOsm/kg i.e., 80 mOsm/kg to a new level of 360 mOsm/kg. Now sodium ion is kept out of the ICF by an active sodium pump extrusion mechanism so that it cannot enter the cells to equalize osmolalities of ICF and ECF. Instead water passes *out* of the ICF *into* the ECF, and so expands the ECF *at the expense* of ICF volume, in order to reduce the change in ECF osmolality. This would require the addition of 1200/280 litres of water from the ICF i.e. 4.285 litres and this in itself would lead to a rise in ICF osmolality. Of course in a healthy man the kidneys would excrete the excess saline by an osmotic diuresis within 3 days. However, before the salt is excreted there will be a degree of expansion of the ECF and some contraction of the ICF.

Question Addition of 600 mEq of sodium chloride to the body causes expansion of:

Answer 1. The ECF Go on to **1.35**.
           2. The ICF. Go on to **1.37**.
           3. Both ECF and ICF. Go on to **1.39**.

1.39   Your answer—sodium chloride enters ECF and ICF.

You are guessing. You should read **1.38** again you will see that ICF has a low sodium content because there is an active sodium pump which extrudes sodium from the cell interior into the ECF. Read **1.38** carefully before choosing the correct answer this time.

1.40   Your answer—congestive heart failure is associated with expansion of ICF volume.

You are wrong. ICF volume does not need to alter. Read **1.35** again with more care this time. Then you will be able to answer this simple question correctly.

1.41   Your answer—in CHF there is an increase in ECF volume.

You are correct. If there is a reduction in water in-take i.e. patients with neglected diabetes mellitus and massive glycosuria, with carcinoma of the oesophagus, in the untended or neglected comatose patient, in diabetes insipidus, shipwrecked mariners, or men stranded in the desert without water, there is an increase in body fluid osmolality all round i.e. in both ECF and ICF, due to loss of fluid from both compartments in the presence of the same amount of solute. Human beings, in the desert for example, can lose up to 12.5 per cent of their body weight as loss of water before they die. Severe dehydration results in their being unable to control their body temperature by sweating, and so then they develop hyperpyrexia and heat stroke. During the development of severe water loss i.e. when they have lost less than 6 or 7 kg there is *no fall* in blood pressure, the pulse rate is not greatly elevated and the patient is not in shock. This is in contrast to the state which ensues if salt *and* water are lost to the body simultaneously. This is considered later. At present you need to remember that the pure water loss is associated with a normal blood pressure and pulse until close to the fatal termination, but the urine is highly concentrated with an osmolality of close to the maximum of 1400 mOsm/kg. This urine concentration is produced by the liberation of vasopressin (antidiuretic hormone) as a result of the perfusion of the osmoreceptors in the hypothalamus by plasma with a higher-than-normal osmolality. Re-read this paragraph.

Now answer the question:

Question In pure water depletion what is the urinary osmolality?

Answer 1. Very high. Go on to **1.45**.
2. Normal. Go on to **1.47**.
3. Low. Go on to **1.49**.

1.42 Your answer—pure water loss.
You are wrong. Go back to **1.48** and read it carefully.

1.43 Your answer—reduction in ECF volume.
You are wrong. Sodium chloride overloading causes an expansion of ECF volume, in which the plasma shares proportionately, leading eventually to congestive heart failure. Re-read **1.35** carefully.

1.44 Your answer—he is suffering from gross ECF volume depletion.
No. You are not reading with adequate concentration. He has no features of dehydration. Read **1.45**, then choose the correct answer in **1.51**.

1.45 Your answer—urinary osmolality is high.
You are correct. If a person loses both sodium chloride and water by vomiting or diarrhoea (such as gastro-enteritis or cholera) or by drainage after an operation, he loses the main constituents of the ECF—sodium, chloride and water i.e. the ECF volume will be reduced. This

reduction occurs in both plasma and interstitial fluid proportionately i.e. 3/15 of the loss is in the plasma and 12/15 in the interstitial fluid. The patient has signs of ECF depletion—fall in blood pressure, first noted as postural or orthostatic hypotension, and later as hypotension in the recumbent position as well; fast thready pulse; loss of elasticity of the skin and reduced eye-ball tension. Bear in mind that in elderly people (65 and over) the skin tends to lose its elasticity somewhat, but this rarely occurs over the sternum and forehead and upper ribs. Remember that the skin of the forearms and the dorsum of the hands are a pons asinorum of apparent loss of elasticity in the non-dehydrated elderly person. Eye-ball tension is reduced so as to be appreciable by the unaided fingers only in very advanced cases of salt and water loss. The ultimate picture is the patient in shock, with Hippocratic facies, thready pulse, unrecordable blood pressure, dry tongue, loss of skin turgor and sunken eyes—all this because of a reduction in ECF volume without change in ICF volume.

Now answer the question:

Question In a patient who has had aspiration of the stomach contents after gastro-intestinal surgery and in whom no fluid replacement of the aspirated fluid has been made, what is the ECF volume?

Answer 1. ECF volume is depleted. Go on to **1.51**.

2. ECF volume is increased. Go on to **1.53**.

1.46   Your answer—pure NaCl loss.

No. You are wrong. You are day-dreaming. Go on to **1.48** and read carefully.

1.47   Your answer—urinary osmolality is normal.

No. Clearly you have no idea of the contents of paragraph **1.41**. You have to concentrate on the contents, unless you wish to waste your time. Go back and read **1.41** again, carefully this time.

1.48   Your answer—he has *no* gross ECF volume depletion.

You are correct. The urine in severe salt and water deficiency may be slightly hypertonic with a urine/plasma osmolality ratio of 1.4 : 1. It may fall to 1.0 : 1 ratio if tubular necrosis ensues. The urine has a low sodium concentration (< 20 mEq/1) unless acute tubular necrosis develops.

Typical causes of massive loss of water and salt simultaneously are pyloric stenosis, severe diarrhoea from gastro-enteritis in infancy and childhood, cholera, staphylococcal entero-colitis, drainage of the gastro-intestinal tract after surgical operations without adequate replacement of the aspirated fluid, drainage of massive quantities of ascitic fluid, and sudden relief of a urinary pathway obstruction by catheterization.

Now answer the question:

Question Cholera causes which of the following?

Answer 1. Pure water loss. Go on to **1.42**.
2. Pure NaCl loss. Go on to **1.46**.
3. Mixed salt and water loss. Go on to **1.61**.

1.49   Your answer—urinary osmolality is low.

You are quite wrong. You have not concentrated when you read **1.41**, so that you produce senseless guesswork answers. Read **1.41** concentrating this time. If you can't concentrate, stop work and do not start again until you have circumstances in which you can concentrate.

1.50   Your answer—statement 3 is false.

You are correct. You may want to read some of the more detailed monographs and original references.

Monographs and Chapters:
1. Brenner B. H. and Stein J. (1978) *Sodium and Water Homeostasis*. Churchill-Livingstone, London.
2. Hays R. M., (1979) Dynamics of body water and electrolytes, in Maxwell and Kleeman's *Clinical Disorders of the Fluid and Electrolyte Metabolism*. Chapter 1, Third Edition. McGraw-Hill, New York.
3. Bland W. H., (1972) Radioisotope techniques, *ibid* Chapter 15.
4. Black D. A. K., (1979) *Essentials of Fluid Balance*, Chapter 2, Fourth Edition, Blackwell Scientific Publications, Oxford.
5. Pitts R. F. (1968) *Physiology of the Kidney and Body Fluids*, Chapter 2, Second Edition. Year Book Publishers, Chicago.
References: Edelman I. S. and Leibman J. (1959) Anatomy of Body water and electrolytes. *Am. J. Med.* **27**, 256.
Windhager E. E. (1969) Kidney, water and electrolytes, *Ann. Rev. Physiol.* **31**, 117.

You can now start Chapter 2 after a rest period.

1.51   Your answer—ECF volume is depleted.
Correct. Now answer the next question. A 70 year old man is suspected of being dehydrated because the skin on the dorsum of his hand is inelastic. The skin over the manubrium sterni is normal. Blood pressure lying and standing is 160/100, and the pulse rate is 64 per minute.

Question Is he suffering from gross ECF volume depletion?

Answer   1. Yes. Go back to **1.44**.
2. No. Go back to **1.48**.

1.52   You are wrong. Statement 3 is wrong. Read the chapter from 1 again.

1.53   Your answer—ECF volume is increased. You are quite clearly not reading with adequate concentration. Read **1.45** again. Then answer the question correctly.

1.54   You are wrong. Statements 1 and 2 are correct. Read the chapter from the beginning again.

1.55   You are wrong. Statement 2 is correct. Read the chapter from the beginning again.

1.56   You are wrong. Statement 1 is correct. Read the chapter from 1 again.

1.57   You are completely wrong. Start the chapter again from the beginning.

1.58   Statement 1 is correct. 3 is false. You should re-read this chapter.

1.59   Statement 3 is false, 2 is correct. Re-read the chapter from the beginning.

1.60   Your answer—demethylchlortetracycline.
You are correct. Now we are coming to a series of questions to test your knowledge to this chapter. Read them carefully then choose the correct answers.

Questions:

Statement 1. ICF volume is greater than ECF volume.
Statement 2. Potassium concentration in ICF is higher than in ECF.
Statement 3. Inulin penetrates all cells.
Which of these statements are correct? Choose the correct answer below.

1. All the statements are correct. Go on to **1.52**.
2. None are correct. Go back to **1.54**.
3. Statement 1 is correct, 2 and 3 are false. Go back to **1.55**.
4. Statement 2 is correct, 1 and 3 are false. Go back to **1.56**.
5. Statement 3 is correct, 1 and 2 are false. Go back to **1.57** .
6. Statements 2 and 3 are correct, 1 is false. Go back to **1.58**.
7. Statements 1 and 3 are correct, 2 is false. Go back to **1.59**.
8. Statements 1 and 2 are correct, 3 is false. Go back to **1.50**.

1.61   Your answer—mixed salt and water loss.
You are correct. Let us look at antidiuretic hormone in more detail.

The posterior hypophyseal hormone, vasopressin, is essential for the maintenance of water homeostasis in man. In the absence of vasopressin, or in conditions where the kidneys are refractory to its action, a condition of diabetes insipidus exists in which the urine concentration is well below that of plasma i.e. the urine is hypotonic. The normal plasma osmolality is 280—285 mOsm/kg whereas urine osmolality in diabetes insipidus is of the order of 150 mOsm/kg, and even in severe dehydration does not rise above that of plasma. In the normal person, however, spot urine osmolalities in the early morning, (after overnight abstention from drinking) are of the order 800—900 mOsm/kg. In diabetes insipidus, you will recall, the urine osmolality is 150 mOsm/kg. Clinically, diabetes insipidus is manifested by severe polyuria as a result of the inability to concentrate the urine in the absence of antidiuretic hormone and an appropriate and possibly exaggerated polydipsia. The renal action of antidiuretic hormone is to stimulate the counter current multiplier system in renal medulla, probably by stimulating actively the extrusion of chloride from the ascending loop of Henle into the interstitium and also enabling water to pass from the tubular lumen of the collecting ducts into the medullary interstitium. The counter current multiplier is not activated in the absence of vasopressin or in cases of renal refractoriness to its action, and so to the osmotic tissue gradient from cortex to papillary tip is much reduced. Hence the urine is not concentrated and urine volume increases to up to 10 or 11 litres a day.

Now answer the question:

Question What is the urine osmolality in untreated diabetes insipidus?

Answer 1. 800 mOsm/kg. Go on to **1.63**.
　　　　　 2. 150 mOsm/kg. Go on to **1.65**.
　　　　　 3. 370 mOsm/kg. Go on to **1.67**.

1.62　Your answer—1 per cent.

No. This is too small a dehydration stress to obtain maximal ADH secretion. Read **1.65** again.

1.63　Your answer—800 mOsm/kg.

No. This answer is the osmolality of spot urine samples taken in the morning in a normal population. You have not achieved the goal of **1.A**. Read **1.61** again.

1.64　Your answer—50 per cent.

No. 50 per cent loss of weight is associated with certain death. 5 per cent is hazardous enough. Read **1.67** again.

1.65　Your answer—150 mOsm/kg.

You are correct. Good. Characteristically, in young children, diabetes insipidus is associated with nocturnal enuresis, but in adults nocturia is predominant, together with nocturnal drinking. Children are often found to be so thirsty that they drink from toilet bowls. If deprived of water they develop hypernatraemia with serum sodium of above 150 mEq/l, and this dehydration due to continued loss of inappropriately dilute urine in the presence of inadequate water intake may result in dehydration of the brain, causing damage to the brain and resulting mental deficiency. This is only of importance in infants, usually male with inherited diabetes insipidus.

Diabetes insipidus is either due to absolute deficiency of vasopressin, or due to insensitivity of the kidney to the action of vasopressin. Let us consider them in more detail.

1. True diabetes insipidus. In this condition of diabetes insipidus there is an absolute or relative absence of the normal amounts of vasopressin in the plasma on stimulation by thirsting. Vasopressin is thus not demonstrable, or demonstrable in very reduced quantity, by bio-assay or radio-immunoassay in the plasma. The urine osmolality is inappropriately low when compared with the plasma osmolality. Diagnosis is made clinically by the low urine osmolality, below that of the plasma, after abstinence from drinking for 24 hours or until the weight loss has reached 5 per cent of the body weight. Never go on longer. It is dangerous.

Question A man weighing 50 kg is put on a 'no fluid' dehydration test to assess his maximal urine osmolality. He is weighed hourly. At what percentage weight loss would you stop the test?

Answer 1. 1 per cent. Go on to **1.62**.
          2. 5 per cent. Go on to **1.66**.
          3. 50 per cent. Go on to **1.64**.

1.66 Your answer: 5 per cent weight loss is maximum.

Correct. Human beings commonly die when there is dehydration resulting in a fall of 12.5 per cent of body weight or more. The camel is more drought resistant and can withstand body weight loss of up to 30 per cent without death. Administration of vasopressin either as lysine vasopressin s.c. or pitressin tannate in oil, 5 units confirms the diagnosis of true diabetes insipidus by the resulting urine osmolality rising well above that of plasma. The conditions leading to diabetes insipidus are trauma, craniopharyngioma and other hypothalamic tumours, meningitis, encephalitis, syphilis and Hand-Schüller-Christian's disease.

2. Renal diabetes insipidus is a disease complex characterized by one common factor— the plasma vasopressin level is normal or raised, but the renal tissues are refractory to its action. Thus the water deprivation test will result in hypotonic urine despite a 5 per cent body weight loss. Also, injection of 5 units pitressin tannate in oil does not cause an increase in urine osmolality. Diseases responsible for renal diabetes insipidus are:

1. Hereditary Renal Diabetes Insipidus, usually sex linked affecting males.
2. Hypercalcaemia.
3. Hypokalaemia.
4. Hydronephrosis.
5. Pyelonephritis.
6. Malignant hypertension (occasionally).
7. Renal Amyloidosis (on occasion).
8. Administration of Demethylchlortetracycline or lithium

Table 1.66   List of antidiuretic drugs (excluding vasopressin and its analogues)

1. Act by stimulation of ADH release
   Barbiturates
   Isoproterenol
   Nicotine
   Morphine
   Vincristine
   Carbamazepine
   Chlorpropamide

2. Act by potentiating small amounts of ADH
   Chlorpropamide
   Acetoaminophen

3. Other actions
   Cyclophosphamide
   Indomethacin
   Tolbutamide

The therapy of true diabetes insipidus is the administration of 1-desamino-8-D-arginine vasopressin—referred to as DDAVP, a synthetic long acting vasopressin, given by nasal drops or spray, or by injection of pitressin tannate. As an alternative chlorpropamide or chlorothiazide can be given. In renal diabetes insipidus chlorpropamide is the drug of choice but care should be exercised due to its hypoglycaemic actions. Chlorothiazide itself may be effective enough to reduce the urine volume to a tolerable 2 or 3 litres a day. Again care should be taken to make sure that its action is not accompanied by urinary sodium loss in excess of dietary salt intake. Look at table 1.66 for other drugs which are antidiuretic. Learn it by heart.

Question What is DDAVP?

Answer 1. An anti-ADH drug. Go on to **1.68**.
2. A synthetic prolonged action vasopressin. Go on to **1.69**.

1.67   Your answer— 370 mOsm/kg.

No. This is a guess. Don't guess. This is supposed to be meaningful learning process where I transfer knowledge from my brain to yours via the printed word. Please concentrate when you read **1.61** again.

1.68   Your answer—an anti ADH.

No. DDAVP is a synthetic analogue of arginine vasopressin of prolonged action. You've missed this. Read **1.66** again.

1.69   Your answer—a synthetic vasopressin.

Good. The syndrome of inappropriate secretion of diuretic hormone (SIADH) was described by Bartter and Schwartz. In this condition antidiuretic hormone is secreted *not in response* to a dehydration stress but paradoxically, resulting in a syndrome of overhydration with water retention and resultant severe hyponatraemia, a low plasma osmolality (well below the normal i.e. plasma hypotonicity) *at a time* when the urine remains hypertonic to plasma. Read this again. Typical findings would be: Serum Na 120 mEq/1, Cl⁻ 80 mEq/1, plasma osmolality 245 mOsm/kg, urine osmolality 500 mOsm/kg. Antidiuretic hormone if given in excess for several days is associated with a sodium leak i.e. urinary sodium loss, so that the low plasma sodium level may reflect not only a dilutional hyponatraemia but also true sodium depletion at least in part.

The causes of inappropriate secretion of antidiuretic hormone include malignant tumours, particularly common being carcinoma of bronchus; chronic infections such as tuberculosis; sarcoid, artificial ventilation; meningitis.

The therapy of SIADH is treatment of the initial disease and also to attack the water retention as follows:

1. To reduce water intake to 500 ml/day and so cause fluid depletion, monitoring the serum sodium level until it rises 135 to 140 mEq/1. Many patients do not keep this regimen.

2. Lithium therapy. Lithium salts causes a diabetes insipidus syndrome and have been advocated for the therapy of SIADH, but its use is not yet established as safe and without hazard.

3. Demethylchlortetracycline in a dose of up to 1200 mg a day will promote a flow of dilute urine, and is at present the therapy of choice.

Question What drug would you use in the therapy of SIADH?

Answer 1. Chlorothiazide. Go on to **1.70**.
           2. Demethylchlortetracycline. Go on to **1.60**.

1.70   Your answer—Chlorothiazide.

No you are confusing therapy of diabetes insipidus and SIADH. Your attention has wandered. Read **1.69** again and concentrate carefully.

Time for this chapter: 2 hours

Chapter 2
Sodium

2.1 Sodium is distributed in the body mainly in extracellular fluid and in the bone. There is a low sodium concentration in the intracellular fluid because of active pumping of sodium *out* of the cells. The cell can be likened to a leaking ship with the pumps working continually to get rid of the water which is seeping in, in order to keep the ship afloat. In the case of the cell the pumps deal with sodium which is seeping passively into the cells *down* a concentration gradient from the high sodium concentration in the ECF to the low sodium concentration inside the cell. Pumping sodium out of the cell requires the expenditure of energy because the movement of sodium is against a chemical concentration gradient. The total amount of sodium in the body is of the order of 5000 mEq for a 70 kg man i.e. $5000/70 = 70$ mEq/kg body weight. The ECF contains about 140 mEq of sodium per litre i.e. 2100 mEq. ICF contains about 10 mEq of sodium per litre i.e. 270 mEq in a 70 kg man. Thus ICF and ECF have a total of about 2370 mEq of sodium, much of the remaining sodium, i.e. around 30 per cent– 40 per cent being in bone. Sodium is present in the lattice of the bone crystals. Much of the bone crystal is embedded deep in the bone and is not in direct contact with ECF.

This inaccessible bone store of sodium is of particular interest when we consider the discrepancies between the various ways available for the measuring of the total body sodium.

Now read the question and choose the right answer.

Question Is there more sodium in the ICF or in the ECF?

Answer 1. In the ECF. Go on to **2.4**.
2. In the ICF. Go on to **2.6**.
3. Don't know. Go on to **2.3**.

2.2 You should not be reading this paragraph. There is no point in reading this book like a normal textbook. You must follow the programme instructions. If you fail to do so there is no guarantee that you will learn from this book; you might as well day-dream over a standard format textbook which is less useful to you.

31

2.3   Your answer—I don't know. Your choice of this answer suggests you don't know the purpose of reading this book. Read the paragraph **2.1** again. If you can't get the correct answer, stop reading for several hours.

2.4   Your answer—more sodium is present in the ECF.

    You are correct. Total body sodium can be measured directly in the human cadaver by incinerating the corpse and dissolving the ashes in mineral acid and then measuring the sodium content of the solution. This has been done on a number of occasions and yields figures which are much higher than isotopically determined exchangeable sodium. Look at this table:

Total body sodium measured chemically in whole cadaver. 57.1 to 67.6 mEq/kg.

Exchangeable sodium (Na_E) determined isotopically. 40.8 to 43.0 mEq/kg.

The total body sodium is greater than isotopically determined or exchangeable sodium (Na_E). To understand why this is we have to know something about exchangeable sodium. Before going on to this, answer the question.

Question   Which is higher, total body sodium estimated chemically or exchangeable sodium?

Answer   1. Total body sodium. Go on to **2.7**.
               2. Exchangeable sodium. Go on to **2.8**.

2.5   Your answer—$Na_E = 45$ mEq/kg. You are correct. Now answer the question:

Question   Is ^{24}Na able to penetrate *all* bone sodium stores in 24 hours?

Answer   1. Yes. Go on to **2.11**.
               2. No. Go on to **2.12**.

2.6   Your answer— more sodium is present in the ICF.

    You are wrong. You have not read **2.1** with adequate concentration. Don't try listening to the radio, records, tapes or watching TV while reading this book. Make sure that you are in quiet surroundings. Then go back and read **2.1** again.

2.7   Your answer—total body sodium is higher.

    You are correct. Now we can go on to discuss exchangeable sodium

Exchangeable sodium (or Na_E) is the term applied to the amount of sodium in the body which exchanges with radioactively labelled sodium either ^{24}Na or ^{22}Na. This is easier to understand if we take the practical example of how exchangeable sodium is measured. The principles of the method are the dilution in the body fluids of a known amount of administered radio-isotopic sodium after an equilibration period of 24 hours: and then measurement of the specific activity of the plasma, urine or saliva at the end of the equilibration period. Specific activity is the number of counts per minute of radioactivity per mEq of stable (non-radioactive) sodium. Thus measurement of the specific activity of plasma sodium 24 hours after radioactive sodium has been given, will give us the dilution of radio-active sodium in the exchangeable pool of stable sodium in the body. Hence we can calculate the amount of stable sodium which has come into equilib-rium with radioactive sodium. This may be difficult for you to follow. Let us look at a typical example of such an experiment.

A 70 kg man receives 250,000 cpm of ^{24}Na, and at the end of 24 hours he has excreted 10,000 cpm in his urine. His plasma contains at this time 140 mEq of sodium per litre and each ml of plasma contains 11.2 cpm. (All counts are measured at the end of the 24 hour period and decay of this short half life isotope, ^{24}Na, is therefore taken into account.)

Total amount of isotope remaining in the body = 250,000 − 10,000 cpm
= 240,000 cpm.

In each *litre* of plasma there are 140 mEq of sodium and 11.2 × 1000 cpm of radioactive ^{24}Na.

Therefore Specific Activity of sodium = 11200/140 = 80 cpm/mEq

Therefore Exchangeable sodium (Na_E) = $\dfrac{\text{Administered radioactivity}}{\text{Specific Activity}}$

$$= \frac{24,000}{80} \text{ mEq}$$

$$= 3000 \text{ mEq}$$

Therefore $Na_E = \dfrac{3000}{70}$ mEq/kg body weight

$$= 42.9 \text{ mEq/kg body weight.}$$

It will be seen that exchangeable sodium of 42.9 mEq/kg is consider-ably less than the total chemically measured body sodium of 70 mEq/kg. The reason for this discrepancy is that much sodium is found in the skeleton in the deeper layers of the bone and therefore 60−75 per cent of

Table 2.7   (Adapted from Mudge 1953)

Total sodium	Wt kg	Na mEq
Whole body	70	5100
Muscle (skeletal)	30	810
Skin	18	1600
Bone	12	1600
Plasma	2.6	363
Liver	1.8	74
Brain	1.9	133

bone sodium does not readily come into equilibrium with the radioactive sodium in the extracellular fluid. In the arterial wall sodium is bound in a mucopolysaccharide complex, and is of importance in the regulation of the sensitivity of the arterial system to pressor drugs.

Look at the table showing the distribution of sodium in the various tissues in man (Table 2.7) note the large amounts of sodium in bone and skin.

Now answer the question:

Question A man weighing 70 kg receives 200,000 cpm of ^{24}Na and excretes 20,000 cpm in his urine in 24 hours. His plasma at the end of this time contains 140 mEq sodium per litre and 8000 cpm/litre. What is his exchangeable sodium, assuming no vomiting or sweat losses or sodium?

Answer   1. 45 mEq/kg. Go on to **2.5**.
            2. 3150 mEq. Go on to **2.10**.

2.8   Your answer—exchangeable sodium is greater.

No you are wrong. Only a certain proportion of sodium is available for exchange. You are not concentrating. Please read **2.4** again. Then answer the question correctly.

2.9   Your answer—Na_E is 3500 mEq/l.

No. You have forgotten to subtract 20,000 cpm lost in the urine, so that the total body load retained is 180,000 cpm. Now the specific activity of sodium is 8000/140 = 57.14 cpm/mEq of sodium, so Na_E = 180,000/57.14 = 3150 mEq.

Therefore $Na_E = \dfrac{3150}{70}$ mEq/kg $=$ mEq/kg.

Read **2.7** again.

2.10 Your answer—$Na_E = 3150$ mEq. You are correct although it is often better to express the result per kilogram of body weight. Thus Na_E is 45 mEq/kg. Go on to **2.5**.

2.11 Your answer—^{24}Na is able to penetrate all the bone sodium stores in 24 hours.
  You are wrong. It is apparent that you have not read **2.7** with adequate attention. Go back and read it again, then answer the question in **2.5** with some more knowledge. If you can't concentrate because of external circumstances or inner turmoil, stop learning for a few hours.

2.12 Your answer—^{24}Na is not able to penetrate *all* bone sodium in 24 hours.
  You are correct. Sodium homeostasis is remarkably efficient. The conservation of sodium is an essential feature of the mammalian body, where sodium is so essential in maintaining the extracellular fluid volume and osmolarity, despite variations in sodium intake which may vary from 700 mEq/l of sodium per day to a virtually sodium free diet. Let us look at the various organs responsible for maintaining sodium balances within such narrow limits.
  Little sodium absorption occurs in the stomach. In the small intestine the absorption of dietary sodium continues pari passu with the absorption of sodium secreted into the gut from the pancreas, bile and the succus entericus. Sodium absorption in the jejunum occurs against a relatively small chemical concentration gradient, and in the presence of bicarbonate there is active transport of sodium. Bulk flow transport in which the passage of water is responsible for the absorption of bicarbonate also occurs. The active transport of sodium in the small intestine is also dependent on the active transport of sugars. By the time the ileum is reached there is a greater gradient with decreasing concentration of sodium in the lumen as the rectum is approached, so that only 1 to 10 mEq of sodium are excreted in the faeces each day, the remaining sodium having been absorbed from the gastro-intestinal contents and excreted in the urine or the sweat. About 50 mEq of sodium are absorbed each day from the colon. The absorption of sodium in the colon is ionically linked to the secretion of

potassium ion, while chloride ion is simultaneously absorbed in exchange for bicarbonate ion.

Now answer the question:

Question   How much sodium is found in normal faeces in 24 hours?

Answer 1. None. Go on to **2.14**.
2. 1–10 mEq. Go on to **2.16**.
3. 10–50 mEq. Go on to **2.18**.

2.13   Your answer—a deficiency of sodium only.

No. In most cases there is also a potassium deficiency. Read **2.16** with more concentration please, and answer the question correctly.

2.14   Your answer—no sodium is found in the faeces.

You are wrong. Don't day-dream. Read **2.12** again, then choose the correct answer.

2.15   Your answer—A deficiency of potassium only.

You are guessing, and not to brightly at that, in view of the subject of the chapter being sodium. Read **2.16** again and concentrate this time.

2.16   Your answer—1–10 mEq/day.

You are correct. The sodium concentration in the faeces is decreased in the presence of aldosterone. Cholera toxin, gastrin and related gastro-intestinal hormones, vasopressin and cyclic AMP are all capable of reducing sodium absorption. Diarrhoea due to malabsorption or any other cause i.e. ulcerative colitis, may lead to massive faecal sodium losses. Pyloric stenosis is of course a common cause of sodium depletion, for not only is the normal dietary sodium intake vomited back, but the vomitus contains substantial amounts of both sodium and potassium ion from the stomach secretions, and their loss commonly causes sodium *and* potassium depletion in cases of pyloric stenosis. Remember to replenish the lost sodium *and* potassium in cases of pyloric stenosis before operation, and so avoid catastrophies on the operating table. Every student of surgery knows that the most rapid sodium depletion may occur in intestinal obstruction just distal to the duct of Wirsung, for then the loss of sodium rich pancreatic secretion is added to the loss of gastric secretion sodium; this loss is less than that in choleraic diarrhoea where the loss of massive amounts of sodium may result in death in a few hours.

Now answer the question:

Question In pyloric stenosis is there a deficiency of sodium, potassium, or both?

Answer 1. Sodium only. Go on to **2.13**.
         2. Potassium only. Go on to **2.15**.
         3. Both Na and K. Go on to **2.17**.

2.17 Your answer—both sodium and potassium are lost.
    You are correct. The renal handling of sodium will now be discussed. Overall the kidney is the main organ responsible for the flexible handling of sodium excretion, depending on the needs of the body. The bowel in health absorbs virtually all sodium presented to it in food, whereas the kidney can excrete varying amounts so as to keep the milieu interieur constant. In practice the kidney excretes 98−99 per cent of the ingested Na in health. Thus the kidney will excrete up to 700 mEq/day if the sodium intake is of this order, and yet if there is no sodium intake then within 4 or 5 days the urine is virtually sodium free i.e. 1−2 mEq of sodium/litre of urine. This remarkable flexibility indicates phenomenal adaptive capability of the mechanism of sodium reabsorption to the prevailing conditions. Let us see how this is mediated. To understand this we will have to learn some renal physiology once again. Most of the sodium filtered in the 180 litres of plasma that pass through the glomerular capillary walls into Bowman's space is reabsorbed. Thus 180 litres of glomerular filtrate are formed each day contain approximately 140×180 mEq of sodium $= 25,200$ mEq. In a normal diet there is 150−200 mEq of sodium, so that this quantity of sodium should appear in the urine of the average man i.e. 200 mEq/day. Thus 25,000 mEq of sodium will be reabsorbed in the renal tubules.
    Expressed as a percentage of the filtered load, reabsorption of sodium is $25000/25200 \times 100 = 99.2$ per cent of the filtered sodium. If a patient is given a low sodium intake, say, in the treatment of hypertension, then the urine-sodium content will fall to 1 to 2 mEq/l in 4 to 5 days. This is indicative of 99.99 per cent reabsorption of sodium. 70−80 per cent of sodium is reabsorbed in the proximal tubule and 10−20 per cent in the distal tubule. Sodium reabsorption in the proximal tubule can be compared to the coarse adjustment of a microscope, doing the crude, lion's share of the work in reabsorption of sodium, irrespective of the needs of the body. The distal tubule including the collecting duct can be likened to the fine adjustment of a microscope, sensitive and varying according to the needs of the body. The amount of sodium reabsorbed by the proximal tubule in

normal health is fairly constant despite varying the intake of sodium between 0 and 300 mEq/day, whereas the distal tubule and collecting duct are ultimately responsible for fine variations of reabsorption of sodium so that sodium balance is maintained.

Now answer the question:

Question What is the normal tubular reabsorption of filtered sodium on a normal sodium intake of 150–200 mEq/day?

Answer 1. 95 per cent. Go on to **2.19**.
2. 99 per cent. Go on to **2.21**.
3. 100 per cent. Go on to **2.23**.

2.18   Your answer—10 to 50 mEq/day.
You are guessing. This book is not a novel, where you can skip a paragraph or two of drivel without losing the plot. You have to read every word. Go back and read **2.12** again, and concentrate.

2.19   Your answer—95 per cent is reabsorbed.
You are incorrect. You would lose so much sodium in the urine that you would soon be sodium depleted. Go back and read **2.17** with concentration, and don't try guessing.

2.20   Your answer–supine hypotension.
No. This develops only after a stage of orthostatic hypotension. You have not read **2.21** with adequate concentration. See if there are external circumstances interfering with your reading, and correct them. If not, stop work for an hour or two and start again on **2.21**.

2.21   Your answer—99 per cent of sodium is reabsorbed.
You are correct. Sodium reabsorption is of cardinal importance to the body to protect the constancy of the milieu interieur. Sodium ion is the major cation of the ECF and therefore is the *major cation contributing to the osmotic pressure of the ECF* and is thus one of the major factors controlling the volume of the ECF. Because of the importance of maintaining homeostasis of the internal environment in renal failure as well as in health, it is wise to examine sodium metabolism in renal failure. Tubular reabsorption of sodium in advanced renal failure is much lower than in health. Let us take the following example. A patient has a GFR of 5ml/min. His diet has 150 mEq of sodium in it, and his weight is stable. His serum sodium is 140 mEq/l. What is his tubular reabsorption of sodium?

Filtered sodium FNa $= \dfrac{5 \times 140}{1000} = 0.7$ mEq/min or 700 μEq/min.

If he has sodium equilibrium, he will excrete sodium in his urine, equivalent to what he eats i.e. 150 mEq/24 hours, give or take couple of mEq in sweat and faeces.

∴   Excreted sodium $= \dfrac{150}{1440} \mu$ Eq/min $= 0.104$ mEq/min $=$

104 μ Eq/min.

Reabsorbed sodium $700-104 = 596$ μEq/min.

Tubular reabsorption of sodium $= \dfrac{\text{Reabsorbed Na}}{\text{Filtered Na}} = \dfrac{596}{900} =$

0.662 or 66.2 per cent.

Can you follow this calculation? Try it yourself.

In a normal person remember that less than 1 per cent of sodium is reabsorbed on the same diet in normal health, whereas in uraemia 33.8 per cent of the filtered sodium was rejected by the tubules at a GFR of 5 ml/min.

The point is that tubular reabsorption of necessity is less in renal failure so that homeostasis can be achieved on a normal diet.

The excessive tubular reabsorbtion of sodium is reduced if the patient is given a diet containing less sodium. This has been recently elegantly reformulated and defined by Bricker. If the patient has a difficulty in tubular reabsorption of sodium (salt-losing nephritis) reduction of salt intake may be dangerous. The volume of the ECF in the presence of normal plasma protein levels, is a major factor determining the plasma volume (you recall that one of the constituent parts of the ECF is the vascular space). Thus a reduced ECF volume in a healthy man will often be accompanied by a reduced plasma volume. An elevated ECF will be usually associated with an increased plasma volume in otherwise healthy persons. Now it is very important that the plasma volume be kept constant in the healthy organism. If it is reduced at first the blood pressure will fall when the patient stands up. This is known as 'orthostatic hypotension'. It occurs because the plasma volume is so low that it prevents the achievement of a normal blood pressure even though there is the maximal vasoconstriction in the lower limbs. At rest in the supine position the plasma volume may be adequate to permit the blood pressure to be within the normal range. If a further reduction of ECF volume occurs i.e. due to more extensive loss of sodium, then the plasma volume may be inadequate to permit a normal blood pressure to be maintained even with the subject lying supine. This is known as *'supine hypotension'*. It is usually accompanied by tachycardia.

Later, as sodium depletion progresses, there is a loss of tissue turgor— the skin over the forearms and upper arms loses its elasticity, so that when lifted up between finger and thumb and released it takes several seconds for the skin fold to fall back and disappear. Later the intra-ocular tension falls, there is a typical hippocratic facies with sunken eyes, and the patient dies in shock with cold nose and extremities, if untreated. The importance of the kidneys in reabsorption of sodium to maintain a constant ECF volume is such *that 6 per cent of the total oxygen consumption of the body is used for this purpose.*

Now answer the question.

Question The first sign of sodium depletion is:

Answer 1. Supine hypotension. Go on to **2.20**.
2. Orthostatic hypotension. Go on to **2.24**.
3. Loss of skin turgor. Go on to **2.22**.

2.22 Your answer—loss of skin turgor.

No. This is a particularly late development. You have not concentrated in reading **2.21**. It is apparent that early sodium depletion is expressed by a minor fall in plasma volume. Go back to **2.21** and read it carefully.

2.23 Your answer—100 per cent.

No. You are guessing. If this were true we would all rapidly die of sodium overload. Don't guess. Concentrate on your work. Read **2.17** again very carefully.

2.24 Your answer—orthostatic hypotension.

You are correct. The sodium content of the body can be reduced by:

1. *Vomiting*: i.e. pyloric obstruction or obstruction of the gastro-intestinal tract where the sodium content of the gastro-intestinal tract secretions and/or pancreatic secretions is lost.

2. *Diarrhoea*: i.e. cholera, staphylococcal gastro-enteritis, ulcerative colitis etc. In a few hours there can be a loss of 10 or more litres of fluid which is sodium containing; this loss results in hypotension, and a fall in ECF and plasma volumes.

3. *Sweating*: in miners and stokers working under conditions of extreme heat and humidity, sweat loss can reach 1 litre/hour containing 17 to 45 mEq of sodium per litre, depending on their degree of acclimatization.
Now answer the question:

Question Why is there hypotension in cholera?

Answer 1. Fall in ECF and plasma volume. Go on to **2.26**.
           2. Sodium depletion. Go on to **2.29**.

2.25   Your answer—1/3 of sodium reabsorbed in proximal tubule.
You are not correct. You have not read **2.29** carefully. Read it again.

2.26   Your answer—a fall in ECF and plasma volume.
You are correct, this being mediated by sodium depletion. Go on to **2.29**.

2.27   Your answer—2/3 of sodium is reabsorbed in the proximal tubule.
You are correct. There is now good evidence to suggest that sodium transport in the loop of Henle is passive and is dependent on the active transport of chloride. The loop of Henle is the principal site of action of the loop diuretics furosemide (Lasix)® and ethacrynic acid (Edocryn)® which inhibit chloride and sodium absorption mainly in this area. Remember this fact. In the distal tubule there are tight junctions between the apical segments of neighbouring tubular cells, that do not permit leaking back of absorbed sodium ions. Remember that the proximal tubule is leaky because the junctions between the apical portions of the proximal tubular cells are not so tight and as a result the proximal tubule is 'leaking' in the sense that sodium ion can leak back *after* absorption and return to the proximal tubular lumen. In contrast to this the distal tubule has very tight junctions so that there is very little leak-back of sodium. The final 10–20 per cent of sodium reabsorption takes place in the distal tubule and the collecting duct. Part of this reabsorption may be in the form of ion exchange, shown in Fig. 2.27 but the bulk of the evidence is in favour of separate systems of secretion of potassium and hydrogen from the distal tubular cell. The evidence for this independence of sodium absorption from potassium secretion in the distal tubule is good and it also appears likely that potassium and hydrogen ion secretion are also separate and independent mechanisms. In the distal tubular fluid under conditions of sodium deprivation, sodium concentration has been found to fall to about 10 mEq/litre.

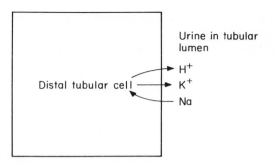

Fig. 2.27

In the collecting duct sodium reabsorption takes place and the final sodium concentration in the urine of a healthy man under conditions of sodium deprivation may fall as low as 1 or 2 mEq/litre. This implies sodium reabsorption against a very large gradient of about 140 mEq/litre, and suggests that this is an active i.e. energy consuming, process.

Sodium reabsorption is under the influence of both mineralocortico-steroids (such as DOCA, aldosterone) and glucocorticosteroids (hydrocortisone); particularly the former enhance sodium reabsorption. Aldosterone is believed to operate by inducing increased synthesis of carrier proteins involved in the sodium pump responsible for sodium reabsorption; in addition vasopressin has a distinct effect decreasing sodium reabsorption i.e. causing an enhancement in sodium excretion. If we want to calculte the amount of sodium delivered to the distal absorption site in man we can do this by assuming that free water (i.e. non-osmotically obligated water) is generated by sodium reabsorption distally. Thus the total amount of sodium delivered to the distal site can be expressed by the formula.

Distal delivered Na = clearance of Na + freewater clearance.

Now answer the question:

Question What is the lowest possible sodium concentration in the urine found 6 days after starting a sodium free diet?

Answer 1. 1 or 2 mEq/l. Go on to **2.30**.
            2. 20 mEq/l. Go on to **2.28**.

2.28   Your answer—sodium concentration of 20 mEq/l.
No. You should realize that it is possible to get a virtually sodium free urine in health, this is stated clearly in **2.27**. Try to concentrate and read **2.27** carefully.

2.29   Your answer—sodium depletion. You are correct. Now we shall consider;

Tubular handling of sodium. Sodium is reabsorbed in the proximal tubule in an isomotic manner i.e. with every litre of glomerular filtrate reabsorbed 140 mEq of sodium are also absorbed. This results in the proximal tubular fluid having nearly the same sodium concentration as the plasma, the difference being due to the Gibbs–Donnan effect. At least 2/3 of the total sodium reabsorption in the kidney takes place in the proximal tubule. The proximal tubular cell has a brush border which increases the area available for absorption many times. The absorption of sodium from the lumen of the proximal tubule is against a small electrical gradient, and thus is an active process and requires energy. The sodium ion is accompanied by the anions chloride and bicarbonate, and there is evidence that rather more bicarbonate and less chloride are absorbed than their relative concentrations in the plasma filtrate. Once sodium gets into the proximal tubule cell, it passes into the intercellular space i.e. the potential space between the cells which interdigitate as

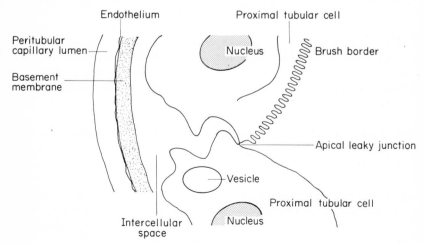

Fig. 2.29

shown in Fig. 2.29. The apical junction is only moderately tight and some sodium can leak back into the lumen.

As sodium accumulates in the intercellular space it attracts water and a vacuole forms in which hydrostatic pressure builds up; the vacuole discharges through the loose basal junction and passes through the peritubular membrane (See Fig. 2.29) into the peritubular space from whence it can be absorbed into the peritubular capillaries. Factors influencing sodium reabsorption in the proximal tubule are (1) a fall in GFR, where less filtrate is formed and therefore less passes into proximal tubule for reabsorption (2) changes in plasma oncotic pressure in the peritubular capillaries. Plasma oncotic pressure is the colloid osmotic pressure exerted in the main by plasma proteins and to a lesser extent by plasma lipids. If the plasma oncotic pressure falls in the peritubular capillaries then there is a decrease in sodium reabsorption from the tubular fluid. Sodium is reabsorbed in the ascending segment of the loop of Henle accompanying active chloride transport and resulting in a hypotonic tubular fluid. Possibly up to 25 per cent of the sodium reabsorbed in the renal tubules is reabsorbed in the loop of Henle.

Now answer the question:

Question In the proximal tubule how much of the total sodium reabsorption takes place?

Answer 1. 1/3. Go on to **2.25**.
2. 2/3. Go on to **2.27**.

2.30 Your answer—1 or 2 mEq/l.

You are correct. The existence of a 'third factor' or natriuretic hormone is difficult either to prove or to refute. There are many substances capable of inducing natriuresis (sodium loss in the urine) including small molecules such as methylguanidine, found in uraemia, as well as large molecules found in uraemic plasma. DeWardener demonstrated the presence of a natriuretic factor in urine but the chemical identification of it has not been made. So far there appear to be several natriuretic hormones of different size and half life which are in the early stages of characterization. In the next few years we may learn more about these. The red cells are suspended in plasma containing a high concentration of sodium, but have very little sodium in them, around 10 mEq/kg of red cells. This implies that there is an active mechanism at work pushing out the sodium which leaks into the red cells from the plasma.

This is the red cell sodium pump, which has the task of continually pumping out the sodium from the cells back into the ECF. This sodium pump is the mechanism for maintenance of a low sodium concentration in the ICF. Similarly in the renal tubule a sodium pump is present for the transport of sodium from the tubular lumen into the cell interior. What is known about the sodium pump? In reality we have a few facts and much theory: The facts are as follows:

(1) There is an enzyme capable of breaking down ATP and dependent on the presence of sodium and potassium ion. This is known as Na, K activated ATPase. The presence of this enzyme is correlated with sodium transport.

(2) The pump can be divided into at least two components in the red cell:

(i) ouabain inhibits sodium efflux from the red cell

(ii) ethacrynic acid or furosemide depresses further ouabain-inhibited sodium efflux.

The metabolic energy for the sodium pump comes from breakdown of energy rich ATP by NaK dependent ATPase in the cell membrane, sodium ion being carried in or out of the cell linked to protein. The enzyme itself is a complex of phospholipid and protein.

Now answer the question:

Question Where does the energy for the sodium pump come from?

Answer 1. From ATP. Go on to **2.32**.
          2. From NAD. Go on to **2.34**.

2.31 Your answer—sodium loss.

You are wrong. How do you come to think you can guess your way through a book like this? Read **2.32** again, this time more carefully.

2.32 Your answer—energy comes from ATP.

You are correct. Plasma sodium levels are held remarkably constant. In health the normal plasma sodium concentration varies from 134 to 145 mEq/litre with mean values for 95 per cent of the examples being 139.7 to 143.7 mEq/litre in males aged 20 to 35 and 137.1 to 143.9 in females. The figures just given are for plasma, and as this contains about 7 g of protein per 100 ml of plasma, the figures need to be corrected if there are large changes in plasma proteins. This means that in patients with dysproteinaemia such as myeloma, the increase in plasma protein concentration decreases the amount of plasma water per 100 ml of plasma; the sodium is mainly in the plasma water, so that a low figure for plasma sodium will result despite a normal concentration of sodium in plasma *water*. This is known as pseudohyponatraemia.

The reverse may be true in patients with hypoproteinaemia where the plasma water content per 100 ml of plasma is increased, and so spuriously high levels of plasma sodium may result although there is no change in the sodium concentration per litre of plasma water. The serum/sodium level is predictably higher than the sodium concentration in lymphatic fluid and interstitial fluid according to the Gibbs—Donnan factor. Loss of sodium from the body is usually accompanied by loss of appropriate amounts of water, so resulting in a reduction in the volume of the ECF with a normal or near-normal serum sodium level. This can be most readily observed as a rapid fall in body weight, then, as the ECF volume continues to contract, orthostatic hypotension appears. This is followed by clinical shock with supine hypotension and a rapid heart rate. In the case of excessive use of diuretics, particularly the loop diuretic frusemide, there is a loss in the urine of sodium but water is still being taken because of thirst and there results a gradual fall in serum sodium concentration to 120 mEq/litre or even less. There may be some accompanying loss of ECF volume but not necessarily so.

Generally a fall in serum sodium i.e. < 130 mEq/l means an excess of water present in the body [e.g. syndrome of inappropriate secretion of antidiuretic hormone (SIADH)] but sometimes actual sodium loss from the body in excess of water loss causes hyponatraemia. The most frequent cause of hypernatraemia i.e. > 150 mEq/l is water deprivation, not excess of sodium in the body.

In pure water loss i.e. not drinking enough to overcome water losses due to causes such as coma, (in which the requirements of the unconscious patient are not being covered by administration of adequate fluids) or in patients who cannot swallow adequately i.e. due to neoplasm of the oesophagus, the serum sodium concentration rises above 147 mEq— to levels of 155 to 160 mEq/l. On rare occasions survival can be observed in spite of dehydration associated with a serum sodium concentration reaching 175 mEq/l.

Rarely hypernatraemia is due to the oral or parenteral administration of massive amounts of sodium salts. Thus in the United States in one outbreak, babies were erroneously given salt in their milk feeds instead of one of the other constituents, and fatalities occured with serum sodium

Table 2.32

Low serum sodium Na < 135 mEq/l	Usually excess water in body; sometimes reduced sodium content in body
High serum sodium > 150 mEq/l	Usually water deficit; very rarely excess sodium

reaching 180 mEq/l. It should be stressed once more that in the *majority of patients* a high serum sodium indicates dehydration.

Look at the Table 2.32. There is some evidence that sodium may enter the cells in excessive amounts under certain circumstances.

(1) When the sodium pump is impaired.
(2) When severe potassium deficiency has reduced cellular potassium concentration, sodium may enter, often accompanied by hydrogen ion.
(3) When intracellular hydrogen ion concentration has fallen, sodium may enter.

Now answer the question:

Question A man is admitted to hospital unconscious following a cerebral haemorrhage. He is found to have a serum sodium concentration of 160 mEq/l. What is the most likely cause?

Answer 1. Sodium loss. Go on to **2.31**.
2. Sodium excess. Go on to **2.33**.
3. Water deprivation. Go on to **2.35**.

2.33 Your answer—sodium excess.

No. Occasionally sodium excess is the cause of a serum sodium of 160 mEq/ l, but this is usually due to the administration of sodium salts, particularly large amounts of intravenous sodium bicarbonate or hypertonic saline. Now go back and read **2.32** again.

2.34 Your answer—the energy for the sodium pump comes from NAD.

No. Stop guessing. NAD is not mentioned at all in **2.30**. This means you have not spent any useful time in reading **2.30**, which goes into the energy dependent sodium pump and discusses what little is known for certain about it. Read **2.30** again.

2.35   Your answer—water deprivation.

You are correct. Now you recall that sometimes hyponatraemia is caused by sodium depletion, rather than excessive water retention. This sodium depletion is associated with a fall in the ECF volume with a reduced plasma volume. The signs are those of ECF volume depletion with plasma volume contraction—increased pulse rate and orthostatic hypotension, later a fall in BP on lying down (supine hypotension), rapid pulse at rest, loss of tissue turgor, fall in intraocular pressure, and vomiting. The urine may be hypertonic as there is release of ADH in response to volume depletion; of course there is also inhibition of ADH release due to the fall in plasma osmolality which accompanies hyponatraemia. Which of these two factors—(inhibition of ADH secretion or stimulation of ADH secretion)—will be effective in any individual case is hard to predict. Certainly as severe contraction of plasma volume occurs it is the rule to find ADH secretion playing a major role in homeostasis, irrespective of the presence of plasma hypo-osmolality.

Hyponatraemia in hypothyroidism. This is a common finding and has been explained as follows:

1. There is a reduction of GFR and less sodium is filtered and brought to the tubular reabsorbing sites: what is brought to the sites is completely reabsorbed, so causing a lowered sodium concentration in the urine and hyponatraemia.

2. There is inappropriate secretion of ADH. This is suggested by a low plasma osmolality with a moderately concentrated urine i.e., a urine osmolality that is much higher than that of plasma.

3. Sodium binding to myxoedema mucopolysaccharides. This is unlikely to account for the hyponatraemia.

4. Low plasma cortisol levels have been implicated. However, these are not usually low in primary myxoedema so that this explanation may only be pertinent in patients with hypothyroidism secondary to hypopituitarism.

Now answer the question:

Question Would you be surprised to find a serum sodium level of 120 mEq/litre in a patient with untreated myxoedema?

Answer   1. Yes. Go on to **2.37**.
          2. No. Go on to **2.39**.

2.36   Your answer—absolute sodium deficit.

You are correct, but you should bear in mind that in view of the hypokalaemia caused by the use of diuretics, sodium may enter the cells and take the place of lost potassium. Now go on to read **2.38**.

2.37   Your answer—yes. I would be surprised.

You are incorrect. If you had read **2.35** properly then you would be quite certain that hyponatraemia occurs in myxoedema, due to either excessive ADH (inappropriate ADH secretion), or sodium binding to myxoedema mucopolysaccharides, or because of low plasma cortisol levels.

Read **2.35** again to find out what else you may have missed out.

2.38   Your answer—sodium has entered the cells in place of potassium.

You are partially correct. But the long term use of diuretics may cause absolute sodium deficit. Remember this fact.

The renin–angiotension–aldosterone system is unique in its contribution to homeostasis of the ECF volume and it does this largely by a servomechanism of dual control involving both blood volume receptors and sodium concentration sensitive receptors in the macula densa of the kidney. There is also some evidence in anephric man of the influence of potassium levels and ACTH on the secretion of aldosterone, where high plasma K stimulates aldosterone secretion. In normal man renin is liberated from the granular cells of the juxta glomerular apparatus in the afferent aterial wall adjacent to the macula densa in response to a fall in arterial pressure or a fall in the sodium content of the macula densa. The renin released is an enzyme which acts on a plasma protein, angiotensinogen, producing a peptide angiotensin I. This is then converted in the blood to angiotension II by a converting enzyme. Angiotensin II is itself vasoactive in very small amounts and is thus used to threat hypotensive shock. Angiotensin II is carried in the blood stream to the zona glomerulosa of the adrenal cortex where aldosterone is released into the adrenal venous blood.

Look at the figure which describes this:

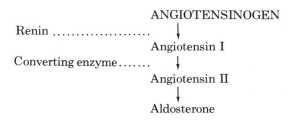

```
                          ANGIOTENSINOGEN
    Renin ....................      ↓
                          Angiotensin I
    Converting enzyme.......      ↓
                          Angiotensin II
                                   ↓
                          Aldosterone
```

There are drugs which block the action of angiotensin II and others block converter enzymes. In hypertension caused by the renin angiotensin system they are variably effective in reducing the blood pressure to normal.

Now answer the question:

Question On what part of the adrenal cortex does angiotensin II act to stimulate the secretion of aldosterone?

Answer 1. Medulla. Go on to **2.40**.
2. Zona glomerulosa. Go on to **2.42**.
3. Zona reticularis. Go on to **2.44**.

2.39 Your answer—no. I would not be surprised.
You are correct.

If a patient is oedematous and hyponatraemic and has hypoprotein-aemia with a low urinary sodium (< 20 mEq/l) it is frequently caused by nephrotic syndrome, or cirrhosis of the liver, or malabsorption. Cardiac failure may also be found associated with a urinary sodium of < 20 mEq/l In hyponatraemic oedematous states in which the urine sodium is elevated greater than 20 mEq/litre the common causes are diuretic administration, and renal failure, either acute or chronic. Look at Table 2.39. Learn it—it is very useful.

In the hypovolaemic hyponatraemic patient it is important to find out whether the hyponatraemia is caused by a renal sodium loss or by non-renal sodium losses. This can be readily ascertained by measuring urinary sodium concentration. If the urine sodium concentration is greater than 20 mEq, then it is likely that a renal sodium loss is present such as RTA, salt losing nephritis, Addison's disease, metabolic alkalosis with bicar-

Table 2.39.   Value of urinary sodium in diagnosis of hypervolaemic (oedematous) patients with hyponatraemia

Urinary sodium < 20 mEq/l	Urinary sodium > 20 mEq/l
1. Nephrotic syndrome	1. Acute renal failure
2. Cirrhosis	2. Chronic renal failure
3. Cardiac failure	

(After Berle and Schrier.)
Learn this table by writing it out 5 times with the book shut.

bonaturia, osmotic diuretics such as glycosuria, or urea osmotic diuresis, and perhaps the most frequent—diuretics. If the urine sodium is less than 20 mEq/litre this indicates an appropriate renal sodium conserving response to the hyponatraemic stimulus. Thus, the cause will be extrarenal, and may be due to gastro-intestinal loss such as vomiting, diarrhoea or ileus; or it may be loss into a 'third space' such as loss in burns—both as exudate into the damaged tissues and loss from the body into dressings; or in muscle damage; peritonitis; and pancreatitis.

Remember that diuretic induced hyponatraemia is usually hypovolaemic but sometimes there is normovolaemia, the sodium having entered cells; administration of potassium will cause the sodium to return to the ECF and plasma sodium levels to normalize.

In Addison's disease there is now good evidence that high plasma levels of ADH are found, and this will tend to exacerbate the hyponatraemia by retention of water; this is helpful in that it blunts the degree of volume depletion associated with the increased urinary sodium loss of hypoadrenalcorticism. In Addison's disease if untreated, hyperkalaemia is usually prominent, the patient having a urine paradoxically rich in sodium and low in K. Clinically the patient is frequently pigmented and has hypotension. The hyponatraemia is not solely due to the sodium leak, for there is an impaired ability to excrete an ingested water load, which is restored to normal by administration of corticosteroids. This test was first described by Dr. S. Oleesky and is often referred to as the Oleesky test. It does *not* differentiate between the impairment of excretion of a water load due to hypoadrenalcorticism and hypopituitarism.

Congestive heart failure is often associated with hyponatraemia. This may be due to excessive use of diuretics causing sodium depletion, but often is associated with water retention or to the occurrence of a potassium deficiency in heart failure, secondary to hypersecretion of aldosterone. There is some evidence that sodium may enter the cells in exchange for potassium lost as a result of the use of diuretics. Look at Table 2.39 again.

ADH potentiating drugs. The sulphonylureas such as chlorpropamide potentiate the action of ADH, as do cyclophosphamide and vincristine. They thus cause a syndrome like that of inappropriate ADH secretion. In Sickle Cell Disease and in the terminal or severely ill patient, of whatever cause, hyponatraemia is often seen as a result of the failure of the sodium pump to get rid of the sodium which leaks into the cells. In cirrhosis of the liver, hyponatraemia may be due to a setting of the osmostat at an abnormally low level with excessive retention of water; the handling of an oral water load may be restored by giving corticosteroids, which may act by increasing the GFR and so causing an increased delivery of sodium to the renal tubules with resultant normalization of sodium and water excretion.

Now answer the question:

Question A patient with severe congestive heart failure for a year due to aortic incompetence has been treated with digoxin and Lasix. His serum sodium level is found to be 118 mEq/l and serum K of 2.5 mEq/litre. What is the most likely cause of the hyponatraemia?

Answer 1. He has absolute sodium deficit due to diuretic use for a year. Go on to **2.36**.
2. He has lost sodium into the cells in place of K. Go on to **2.38**.

2.40 Your answer—medulla. Since when is the medulla part of the adrenal cortex?

You are not working properly. Read **2.38** again, and pay attention to every word. Learning is not easy, but once you have learned something it is a real achievemment.

2.41 Your answer—statement 1 is true, 2 and 3 are false.

You are wrong. This is a short chapter and you should read it again.

2.42 Your answer—Zona glomerulosa.

You are correct. Aldosterone acts on both proximal and distal renal tubules, the intestine, sweat and salivary glands causing a reabsorption of sodium in exchange for potassium which is secreted. β blockers such as propanalol (Inderal®) diminish renin secretion; angiotensin II levels have a feedback type of control on renin levels, so that when angiotensin II is infused i.v., renin levels fall. This type of feedback mechanism is frequently found in the endocrine system and it ensures adequate and efficient control of angiotensin II levels. Potassium depletion stimulates renin secretion, and potassium loading depresses renin secretion. When there is sodium depletion renin levels are increased; in states of sodium repletion, renin levels are depressed. In salt-depleted man there is a reduction in sensitivity to the pressor effect of angiotensin II. The delay in the effect of intravenously injected aldosterone on sodium transport in the renal tubule, gastro-intestinal tract, sweat and salivary glands, has been attributed to the action of aldosterone being to stimulate the synthesis of a protein component of the sodium pump, or of an enzyme, permease, which facilitates the passage of sodium across the cell membrane. Primary hyperaldosteronism is a rare disease in which an adenoma, hyper-plasia or carcinoma of the adrenal cortex produces excessive quantities of aldosterone giving rise to hypertension with hypernatraemia, and hypo-kalaemia. Hypernatraemia is rare in secondary hyperaldosteronism secondary to such conditions as renal artery stenosis, hypoproteinaemia, congestive heart failure, renal failure, hepatic cirrhosis, and diuretic therapy.

In severe hypertension there is frequently a high plasma aldosterone level with high or normal plasma renin levels but in primary aldosteronism plasma renin levels are usually depressed. Low plasma renin levels as-sociated with low plasma aldosterone levels in hypertension are suggestive of another steroid being responsible such as 18 hydroxydeoxy-corticoster-one (18 OH DOC) which suppresses the renin response.

Hyperkalaemia is a frequent finding in hyporeninic hypoaldosteron-ism, a condition found with low renin and aldosterone levels and hyper-kalaemia, most commonly in diabetics. It responds well to fludrocortisone and diuretics.

Retention of sodium and hypokalaemia may also be found in liquo-rice addicts. Renin secreting tumours caused by renal haemangioperi-cytoma are very rare, and are associated with hypertension, hyponatraemia, alkalosis, and high renin and aldosterone levels.

Now answer the question:

Question Is hypernatraemia common or rare in hyperaldosteronism secondary to renal artery stenosis?

Answer 1. Rare. Go on to **2.45**.
2. Common. Go on to **2.47**.

2.43 Your answer—statement 2 is true; 1 and 3 are false.
You are wrong. Go back and read this chapter again.

2.44 Your answer—zona reticularis.
No. You are confusing the layers of the cortex, or you are guessing. You should remember that the glomerulosa is the site of aldosterone production. Read **2.38** again.

2.45 Your answer—hypernatraemia is rare in secondary aldosteronism.

You are correct.

Renal salt wasting due to mineralcorticoid defect is found in hypoadrenalcorticism (Addison's disease) due to idiopathic causes, tuberculosis, amyloid or surgical removal of the adrenal glands as in patients with breast cancer. Sodium depletion with hypercalcaemia is characteristics of this condition. Low plasma cortisol levels and a defect in excretion of an ingested water load with restoration of water load excretion after administration of hydrocortisone are hallmarks of hypoadrenalcorticism.

In adrenogenital syndrome in infants there is an enzyme defect either in the more common 21 hydroxylation defect or the less frequent 3β hydroxyldehydrogenase defect, resulting in defective cortisol production and excessive formation of DOC and corticosterone; if aldosterone formation is blocked some of these children exhibit salt wasting with excessive loss of sodium in the urine. Prostaglandins A_2 and E_2 α have naturiuretic properties associated with impaired renal tubular sodium reabsorption and an increase in renal blood flow. They appear to be implicated in the pathogenesis of Bartter's Syndrome where there is severe hypokalaemia, high aldosterone levels and normal BP. It partially responds to the prostaglandin synthetase inhibitor—indomethacin.

In the majority of chronic renal failure patients hypertension can be controlled by adequate depletion of sodium. In some however, there is an excessive amount of renin produced; renin production is stimulated even further by further sodium depletion; consequently hypertension is exacerbated. This is an unusual response to sodium depletion. There is usually a very adequate response to β blocking drugs such as propanolol which, despite the status of the sodium household (i.e. the amount of sodium in the body) cause a fall in plasma renin levels and a fall in blood pressure.

Now answer the question.

Question Does salt wasting occur in some cases of adrenogenital syndrome?

Answer   1. Yes. Go on to **2.49**.
       2. No. Go on to **2.51**.

2.46 Your answer—statement 3 is true, 1 and 2 are false.

You are wrong. Go back to the beginning of the chapter and read it again.

2.47   Your answer—hypernatraemia is common in secondary aldosteronism.
 You are wrong. You should re-read **2.42** before answering the question.

2.48   Your answer—all the statements are true.
 You are wrong about statement 2. Go back and read the chapter again.

2.49   Your answer—Yes—salt wasting does occur.
 You are correct. Let us have another look at:

Hyponatraemia.   TA reduction in ECF volume, if particularly severe, will result in a massive fall in plasma volume to such an extent that the neck veins do not fill even when the patient lies supine. Other causes of such a loss of blood volume are hypoproteinaemia (usually hypoalbuminaemia) and blood loss i.e. haemorrhage. These must always be excluded in any patient with a reduced plasma volume. In hypovolaemia due to contraction of the ECF caused say, by sodium depletion, or due to hypoproteinaemia or bleeding, there is an increase in tubular sodium reabsorption and in bicarbonate reabsorption. There is a fall in the total ECF volume but the total amount of bicarbonate in the ECF is unchanged, so that with ECF volume reduction the plasma bicarbonate concentration rises. This gives rise to the so called 'contraction alkalosis'.

Therapy of hyponatraemia and dehydration: if the patient has hyponatraemia with a contracted plasma volume it is imperative to replace the plasma volume as soon as possible by means of intravenous saline solutions. If there is obvious hypotension then i.v. normal saline should be infused. It is all very well to define the amounts of salt and water to be infused by 'theoretical' considerations based on dubious guess work cloaked as sacred facts. We advise the pragmatic approach which is used by most physicians engaged in day to day therapy of patients with electrolyte disorder. Let us look at ECF volume contraction. Therapy is based on the following principles: 1. Make a rough estimate of the loss of body fluid in kilograms if one is fortunate enough to know the normal weight of the patient, as well as the present weight of the patient. One must insist on bed scales to determine the weight of the unconscious or bedridden patient. *The loss or gain in body weight in a few hours or days is predominantly body water.* One can conclude from the presence of hyponatraemia that Na^+ has either been lost from ECF *into* the ICF or

has been lost from the body entirely. It is nice to be able to differentiate between these 2 groups, but not always possible in the clinical
situation.

It is therefore wise to replace fluids in these patients empirically with
i.v. saline 0.9 per cent, a litre, rapidly over the 1st hour to 2 hours if
there is supine hypotension or other evidence of gross reduction of intravascular volume. To be sure that there is neither undertreatment (with its
danger of reduced organ perfusion, and renal failure), nor overtreatment
(with its danger of congestive heart failure) it is wise to have continuous
monitoring of vital signs during the infusion—pulse rate, blood pressure
and central venous pressure, and, if possible a pulmonary wedge pressure
with a Swan–Ganz catheter. Most house officers can insert a venous
infusion and measure central venous pressure. Insertion of Swan–Ganz
catheters for measuring pulmonary wedge pressures, needs more expert
handling and there may be some difficulty in obtaining pulmonary wedge
pressures instantly in many hospitals. Often there is a wait of one or
more hours while the patient is transferred to the intensive care unit, the
Swan–Ganz catheter passed, its position verified by X rays and its connection to the transducers for pressure measurements. The aim of therapy
is to restore plasma volume rapidly and safely towards normal, so this can
be monitored clinically by observing the rise in supine blood pressure to
normal levels, a fall in tachycardia to normal pulse rates and normalization of central venous pressure.

Central venous pressure in the dehydrated patient may be zero, and
the aim should be to gently push the i.v. fluids as CVP rises to 14 cm
H_2O. It is best to be on the safe side and not let CVP go above 16 cm
H_2O, so as to avoid overhydration where the CVP may still be normal
with a pulmonary wedge pressure of 25 mm. This enables one to stop over-
hydrating the patient and prevent morbidity and mortality. If there is a
Swan–Ganz catheter in the dehydrated patient a zero wedge pressure
may be found but it will rise on rehydration to 6 mm Hg, and it is wise not
to further push fluids. The major advantage of the pulmonary wedge pressure over central venous pressure is in patients with right sided valvular
heart disease and in pulmonary disease patients, as well as in those
acutely developing left ventricular failure. In the presence of hypoalbuminaemia the CVP or pulmonary wedge pressure may not rise
although too much saline has been administered, because of the low plasma
oncotic pressure which will permit the ECF to expand without any increase
in intravascular volume. This is seen clinically as oedema, pleural
effusions, anasarca and ascites. Thus in patients with known hypoalbu-

minaemia the attempted correction of ECF contraction with saline infusions can result in the formation of oedema and effusions.

Therefore in these patients *hypoalbuminaemia should be corrected first* by the administration of albumin or plasma intravenously. It is not wise to give more than 50 g of albumin i.v. in any 24 hour period lest the serum oncotic pressure rise so far that a massive rise in plasma volume occurs and heart failure supervenes. Careful monitoring of the central venous or pulmonary wedge pressures will prevent over infusion of albumin. *The message is: monitor BP, pulse, CVP/or Pulmonary Wedge Pressure whenever correcting dehydration so as to prevent over or under-treatment.* Learn it and do it. You will save lives by this careful approach.

Question A patient has a serum albumin of 2.0 g/100 ml due to Crohn's disease. He has become dehydrated from severe diarrhoea, with BP on standing of 70 systolic, and a supine BP of 110/70. His CVP is 1 cm of water. What solution would you first give him to replenish his plasma volume?

Answer 1. Saline 0.9 per cent. Go on to **2.55**.
          2. Albumin. Go on to **2.57**.
          3. Dextrose 5 per cent. Go on to **2.59**.

2.50 Your answer—statement 1 is false.
No. You have not retained the material. Go back and read through the chapter again.

2.51 Your answer—salt wasting does not occur in adrenogenital syndrome.
You have not been paying attention to the paragraph you have just read. Either remove the distraction from the environment or go and learn in a quieter place. Read **2.45** again.

2.52 Your answer—statement 2 is false.
You are correct. If you want to read more on sodium I would recommend Swales book on *Sodium Metabolism*, published by Lloyd-Luke, 1975. There are useful chapters in Maxwell and Kleemans *Clinical Disorders of Electrolytes and Body Fluids*. The most up to date book is *Sodium and Water Homeostasis*, edited by B. H. Brenner and J. Stein, 1978, Churchill Livingstone, London. Now go on to Chapter 3.

2.53 Your answer—statement 3 is false.

No. You have not retained the material in this chapter. Read it again.

2.54 Your answer—all statements are false.

This is wrong. You have not learned the material in the chapter. Go back and learn it carefully.

2.55 Your answer—give 0.9 per cent saline first.

No. This would result in an increase of ECF in the extra vascular compartment but no increase in the ICF volume because the low serum albumin reduces the plasma oncotic pressure. Read **2.49** again. You have not read it carefully enough.

2.56 Your answer—yes I would give 1 litre of 5 per cent saline in 1 hour.

You are wrong. 1 litre of 5 per cent saline contains over 850 mEq/1. This is about one quarter of the total exchangeable sodium in the body. Do you think it is wise to give such a load i.v. in 1 hour? Obviously it is potentially lethal. Read **2.57** again—this time carefully, please.

2.57 Your answer—give albumin first.

Correct. We have pointed out that the quantity of fluid to be given should at most equal the weight lost, and that probably in practice this may be less, depending on the response of the servo-mechanism of blood pressure, pulse rate and CVP or pulmonary wedge pressure. Obviously the urine volume, and continuous loss of fluids from other sources i.e. nasal tube, drainage tubes, insensible loss in sweat and via respiration, have to be taken into account in replacing fluid. Also add 100 ml/day per °C (about 60 ml/°F) of fever.

What should be the composition of the fluid to be infused? This depends on the electrolyte abnormality as reflected in the plasma electrolyte picture. If there is a massive loss of sodium and water with or without hyponatraemia it is probably wisest to give normal saline (0.9 per cent NaCl). If there is an acidosis Hartman's solution or Ringer Lactate should be avoided because of the danger of lactic acidosis, it is better to add sodium bicarbonate 1 ampoule (45 mEq) per litre of saline.

If there is a renal failure of hyperkalaemia, then do *not* give potassium containing fluids such as Hartman's solution. It is wisest to use simple solutions without eponyms. The question of hypertonic saline i.e. 3 or 5 per cent NaCl with or without diuretic is frequently raised by house staff in the treatment of hyponatraemia. Generally hypertonic saline should be considered a potentially lethal therapy in amateur hands. It should only be given by a nephrologist of experience. Why is this? Let us look at 5 per cent NaCl. It contains about 860 mEq Na per litre so that if 1 litre is given it may draw into the ECF up to 6 litres of extra fluids, i.e. from ICF, and potentially cause heart failure. Obviously if the patient is severely sodium depleted this extra 6 litres pulled out of the cells may be just what the patient needs, but bear in mind that the hypertonic saline can be dripped in mindlessly by any nurse in an hour and kill the patient very rapidly from heart failure due to EFC expansion, whereas it is very unlikely that 6 litres of normal saline will ever be dripped in the course of 1 hour, without nursing staff noticing that they have to change the litre bottles every 10 minutes which will cause them to question you. This is an intrinsic safety device which is built into the use of normal (0.9 per cent) saline and which is absent in the use of hypertonic saline. If nevertheless you want to use hypertonic saline, then never give more than 250 ml in 3 to 6 hours, and monitor vital signs including BP, pulse rate, neck veins, CVP, pulmonary wedge pressure, absence of crepitations at the lung bases, and absence of oedema. Get serum electrolyte figures $\frac{1}{2}$ to 1 hour after each 250 ml of hypertonic saline has been run in and proceed slowly. Remember to watch patients on hypertonic saline very closely.

What are the indications for the giving of half normal saline? When the patient is losing fluid through any pathway (urine, suction, diarrhoea and drains) with a sodium content of around 70 mEq/l, then give half normal saline. This is conveniently prescribed as 500 ml of 0.9 per cent saline followed by 500 ml of 5 per cent dextrose solution i.v., i.e. equivalent to 1 litre of 0.45 per cent saline.

Question Would you prescribe a litre of 5 per cent saline over a period of 1 hour for a patient with sodium depletion?

Answer 1. Yes. Go on to **2.56**.
            2. No. Go on to **2.58**.
            3. Don't know. Go on to **2.60**.

2.58 Your answer—no. I would not give 1 litre of 5.0 per cent NaCl in 1 hour.

Correct. Remember the golden rule in i.v. electrolytes: *maintain the ECF composition constant*. If we can measure electrolyte losses from all sources and replace them with an equal amount of the same electrolytes in the volume of fluid we calculate to be necessary, then the ECF will automatically have a constant composition in the absence of renal failure. Read this again. Obviously if the ECF were grossly abnormal in quality and in ionic composition then this would need to be corrected by giving fluids of appropriate composition. An example of this would be a patient who has hyperkalaemia—say plasma K was 6.5 mEq/l. Potassium should not be included in his replacement fluids until the plasma K level had dropped to normal. If he has renal failure electrolyte management is more complex but the frequent use of the artificial kidney can prevent gross electrolyte abnormalities developing in even the hypercatabolic anuric patient with the most complicated electrolyte picture. The volume of fluid to be given to a patient is calculated as follows:

1. All fluid losses—vomiting, diarrhoea, urine, surgical drains and gastric suction, are added up daily.
2. Add to this 100 ml for each °C rise in body temperature above 37°C (about 60 ml/°F above 98.4°F).
3. Add 500 ml of a normal sized adult. You know of course that this 500 ml is less than the litre of insensible loss i.e. loss through the lungs in expired air and insensible sweating which adds up to about 1 litre a day in the healthy 70 kg adult. However, there is *production* of water in the body *water of metabolism* (i.e. breakdown of fats, carbohydrates and proteins yields water) *plus the water liberated by the natural breakdown of cells*: these add up to 500−600 ml/day. Obviously the precise amount varies according to the metabolic rate of the patient; losses through the skin and burned areas in patients suffering from burns are immense, and are dealt with in a special section later on (Chapter 8).

Let us look at an example of the fluid replacement calculation. A man with post-operative acute renal failure following septicaemia after colectomy passes 200 ml of urine (sodium content 50 mEq/l); the drain from his abdomen leaks a fluid containing 100 mEq of Na/l and his total loss through the drain is 500 ml/day. His nasogastric tube yields 3 litres with 70 mEq of Na per litre. He has a temperature of 102°F. How much fluid and sodium does he need? The answer is as follows:

A. Fluid volume
1. Fluid loss = 200 ml (urine) + 500 ml (drain) + 3000 ml (nasogastric) + 240 ml (fever loss) = 3940 ml.

Give 3940 + 500 ml = 4400 ml in the next 24 hours. The 500 ml just added to 3940 comes from the net insensible loss.

B. Sodium loss

in urine $= \dfrac{200 \times 50}{1000} = 10$ mEq

in drainage fluid $\dfrac{500 \times 100}{1000} = 50$ mEq

in nasogastric tube 3 × 70 = 210 mEq

Total loss = 270 mEq.

The 270 mEq can be replaced as follows: Normal (0.9 per cent) saline contains 155 mEq/litres therefore the patient should be given 1.74 litres of 0.9 per cent saline and 4.44−1.74 litres of dextrose 5 per cent (DSW) i.e. 2.7 litres of dextrose 5 per cent (DSW).

This will maintain his sodium and water balance. In practice we would give 1.75 litres of N saline over 6 hours and the remaining 2.7 litres of dextrose 5 per cent (DSW) over the remainder of the 24 hours. Go over the calculation again.

Question A post-operative ileus patient loses 2000 ml per day from the nasogastric tube, is apyrexical, urine volume 1200 ml. What fluid volume does he need per day?

Answer 1. 3200 ml. Go on to **2.61**.
2. 3700 ml. Go on to **2.63**.
3. 1000 ml. Go on to **2.65**.

2.59 Your answer—Give dextrose 5 per cent.
No. The dextrose 5 per cent will only add to total body water; it will not expand the ECF specifically and the plasma volume in particular. You have not read **2.49** adequately. Read it again.

2.60 Your answer—I don't know.
Use your mind and spend your time reading and concentrating. In **2.57** a great deal is said about hypertonic saline, 1 litre of 5 per cent saline contains about 850 mEq. This is about 1/4 of the exchangeable sodium in the body. Is it wise to give this i.v. in an hour? Obviously not. You are not even guessing correctly. Go on to read **2.57** again.

2.61   Your answer—3200 ml.

No. You have forgotten to add in the insensible loss minus the water of metabolism and cell destruction. Read **2.58** more carefully.

2.62   You should not be reading this. You are not following instructions.

2.63   Your answer—3700 ml.

You are correct. What if a patient is hypernatraemic—say plasma Na 165 mEq/1? Hypernatraemia in most cases means water deprivation; in a few cases it is due to an actual excess of sodium in the body due to sodium containing drugs or i.v. sodium bicarbonate, but this should be apparent from the history and the prescription sheet on his chart. If there is an absolute excess of sodium—and remember this is rare—a diuretic and oral water or i.v. dextrose 5 per cent will correct it slowly i.e., frusemide 80 mg i.v. and 4 litres of dextrose over the next 12 to 24 hours. If the patient is truly water depleted and has a functioning intact gastro-intestinal tract then water should be given, either by nasogastric tube, or drinking (if he is capable of swallowing) at a rate of a litre per hour for 4 hours, with hourly monitoring of serum sodium levels. This provides the essential feedback to govern the rate and amount of fluid to be given. If the patient is unable to swallow, then give the fluid as i.v. dextrose 5 per cent (DSW). It is necessary to lower the serum sodium moderately quickly to avoid the brain being damaged by a leaching out of water from the brain cells into the hyperosmotic hypernatraemic plasma and interstitial fluid, so that 1 litre per hour of 5 per cent dextrose for the first 4 hours may be necessary. Let us look at the serum Na level at hourly intervals to make sure that we are not going too slowly. Once the serum Na has reached a safe level, say 150 mEq/litre, proceed much more slowly with the i.v. fluid because we do not want to lower the ECF osmolality excessively and go from the shrunken brain cells of hypernatraemia to the cerebral oedema of hyponatraemia, where fluid enters the cells to lower the intracellular osmolality. This can only happen once we have passed the stage of normalization of hydration of the cerebral cells, and should not occur if the last 5 mEq/litre of excess plasma sodium i.e. 150 to 145 mEq/litre are *slowly* corrected.

When you are giving i.v. fluid make sure that you write up your instructions clearly; that vital signs including CVP are carefully monitored; and that you have both a clinical and biochemical feedback.

Never give all the theoretical requirements of fluids in one rapid infusion, but space it out over a 24 hour period, and check the electrolytes in the critically ill patient on i.v. fluids at least once a day when he is in an unstable condition. Learn this. It is very important.

Question Would you rely solely on your theoretical calculations in giving i.v. electrolytes, or would you prefer to have frequent electrolyte results and clinical monitoring to help guide you?

Answer 1. Theoretical calculations are enough. Go on to **2.64**.
2. Electrolyte and clinical monitoring. Go on to **2.66**.

2.64 Your answer—theoretical calculations are enough.

No. This is a most dangerous attitude, and only justified if you are working in primitive conditions where neither laboratory nor clinical monitoring are available, I doubt whether clinical monitoring is *ever* impossible. Read **2.63** again and think about it.

2.65 Your answer—1000 ml. No. That is pure guesswork. Go back and read **2.58** again, this time carefully. Don't try to fool yourself.

2.66 Your answer—both electrolyte and clinical monitoring.
You are correct.

Treatment of oedema. Oedema is an expression of an increase in ECF either locally or generally. Local oedema may be caused by an increase in venous pressure causing an increased exudation of fluid *from* the capillaries *into* the interstitial space, as occurs with venous occlusion i.e. thrombophlebitis. More widespread or generalized oedema may be caused by renal retention of sodium and water with resulting ECF expansion. It is a general rule that an adult weighing 70 kg initially needs to retain a further 4 kg of ECF before oedema becomes apparent. The causes of oedema are shown in Table 2.66. Learn it.

The sodium retention which causes oedema may be stimulated by heart failure or may be due to a fall in the serum proteins. Occasionally there are other, rarer causes. The pathogenesis of oedema goes through an identical common pathway in all causes of oedema other than local venous obstruction. This common pathway is the stimulation of aldosterone secretion so that there is maximal tubular sodium reabsorption, the urine becomes virtually sodium free i.e., 1–2 mEq of sodium per litre. Water is also osmotically obligated by the retained sodium; thus for every 140 mEq of sodium, a litre of water is retained i.e., the weight of the patient goes up by 1 kg. This is because the sodium concentration of ECF

Table 2.66.   Causes of oedema

(a) Local	Increased venous pressure	Phlebitis, thrombosis, pressure from external causes—gravid uterus, tumours, lymph nodes, trauma.
	increased lymphatic pressure	Inflammatory, lymphoedema, malignant lymph gland obstruction, extirpation of lymphatics surgically, e.g. post radical mastectomy, elephantiasis due to filarial infection.

(b) Generalized

I. Raised Venous Pressure
1. Congestive heart failure.
2. Constrictive pericarditis.

II. Lowered Plasma Oncotic Pressure
1. Nephrotic syndrome.
2. Cirrhosis of liver.
3. Malabsorption syndromes, e.g.:
    1. Short bowel post-op
    2. Tropical sprue
    3. Short circuit ops for obesity
    4. Coeliac disease (childhood, adult)
    5. Crohn's disease
    6. Giardiasis
    7. Ellison-Zollinger
    8. Pancreatic disease
    9. Obstructive jaundice
    10. Post-gastrectomy
4. Malnutrition—protein/calorie—(Kwashiorkor)

III. Endocrine
1. Premenstrual oedema
2. SIADH with sodium excess intake.
3. Pregnancy
4. Cyclic (idiopathic) oedema in women

IV. Renal Failure—with ingestion of water and sodium beyond the kidney's ability to excrete it.

Learn this Table, then write it out 5 times with the book closed.

is about 140 mg/1. If you know the weight increase and the serum sodium level you can hazard a fairly accurate guess as to the amount of sodium retained. The urine becomes virtually sodium free under maximal aldosterone stimulation unless large amounts of vasopressin are present when sodium escapes into the urine. This is known as vasopressin mediated 'sodium escape'. This is important in the syndrome of inappropriate antidiuretic hormone (vasopressin) secretion (SIADH) when the ECF volume may be so expanded as to cause oedema but in which the urine is not sodium free.

The stimulus to aldosterone secretion in oedema forming patients is either a reduced vascular volume, stimulating renin release in the kidney, as is found in hypoproteinaemia of any cause, or an increased central venous and right heart volume as is found in congestive heart failure. The renin acts on the adrenal cortex and causes the release of aldosterone which results in enhanced sodium reabsorption in the renal tubuli. The reabsorbed sodium retains osmotically obligated water with it so that for every 140 mEq of sodium retained there must be a litre of water retained. Thus the patient's weight goes up about 1 kg for every 140 mEq of sodium retained. These simple physiological facts give immediate insight into methods of prevention of oedema and its therapy.

Prevention of oedema formation. 1. Dietary methods. A sodium free diet, if the patient can tolerate it, will result in a cessation of the accumulation of oedema. If no sodium is being taken in, none can be retained as oedema. However few diets are entirely sodium free, and those which are—such as the Kempner Rice Diet—are very difficult to keep for a long period of time. If we take more readily available diets, then a 10 mEq Na diet is difficult to adhere to (one needs low sodium milk and low sodium bread), but a 25 mEq Na diet is more practicable. One can stick to such a diet with a little difficulty—it may under maximal aldosterone secretion conditions cause at the most a gain of 1 kg of oedema in 140/25 days i.e. in 6 days even if the patient is anuric. Diets with more sodium will potentially cause a greater ECF retention.

Question How much weight should be gained if 280 mEq of sodium are retained as oedema?

Answer 1. 1 kg. Go on to **2.67**.
2. 2 kg. Go on to **2.69**.
3. 3 kg. Go on to **2.71**.

2.67 Your answer—1 kg.
No. You have not read **2.66**. Read it again.

2.68 Your answer—Yes.
This is not correct. The danger of aldactone in renal failure is hyper-kalaemia. Read **2.69** again.

2.69 Your answer—2 kg. You are correct.

Therapy of oedema. This diet alone is not enough to treat oedema. At the best a diet low in Na can maintain the *status quo* in sodium balance. Therefore one is obliged to get rid of sodium from the body by use of diuretics as well. The commonly used diuretics are the thiazides, and the very powerful loop diuretics such as furosemide. Thiazides are cheap, and less potent than loop diuretics. They should be used first and one can always go on to the use of frusemide if they fail. The dose of chlorothiazide to be given is 0.5 g b.i.d. initially or t.i.d. It is best not given in the evening so that the patient has sleep undisturbed by the need to pass large amounts of urine. The patients should be weighed daily to determine whether ECF has been lost i.e., to see whether the diuretic is successful in removing sodium and fluid. The patient *must* be on a limited sodium intake i.e. 50 mEq/day, so that the diuretic has a chance of causing a loss of more sodium in the urine than is being taken in by ingested diet. Also one must make sure that sodium is *not* being taken in an occult form of medicine i.e. saline i.v., sodium bicarbonate, Kay-exalate (Resonium A), sodium containing purgatives such as sodium sulphate. A 50 mEq sodium intake is relatively easy to keep, and diuretic therapy should be able to maintain a negative sodium balance (i.e. greater than 50 mEq/ day in the urine) if properly managed in most patients. In some patients the thiazides are insufficient and frusemide may be used instead, starting with 40 mg initially or a stronger thiazide, metolazone may be needed, in a dose of 5 mg b.d.

Larger doses are needed in renal failure (0.5 g, b.i.d. or t.i.d.). The addition of spironolactone (Aldactone A®) in a dose of 25 mg q.i.d. may be helpful if there is no renal failure—otherwise the danger of using this aldosterone antagonist may be considerable because hyperkalaemia may develop in renal failure patients treated with aldosterone antagonists. Most diuretics have the same draw-backs in treating oedematous non-uraemic patients i.e. they cause hyperuricaemia, reduced glucose toler-ance resulting in diabetes mellitus and hypokalaemia. Tienilic acid is the only uricosuric diuretic on the market today. Hypokalaemia is rarely a problem but can be treated or prevented by oral potassium supplements, either in the form of dried fruits, bananas and french fries (chips) or as oral supplements as slow K, each tablet having 8 mEq of K. All oral potassium chloride tablets cause some degree of small intestinal ulceration, dried fruits and foods appear to be a safer and more pleasant method of overcoming the danger of prolonged loss of potassium in the urine. These methods together then—diuretics +low salt intake +aldosterone antagonists will get rid of oedema in most patients. In some patients particularly cirrhotics this is not so, and oedema is resistant to diuretics. In these patients there is usually a sodium diuresis when a Le Veen shunt is inserted—this is a valved tube connecting the peritonal cavity with the subclavian vein. Never use spironolactone or triamterene in renal failure. They may cause fatal hyperkalaemia.

The response to the Le Veen shunt is dramatic. The ascites rapidly disappear. An alternative and equally brilliant but non-invasive and purely temporary therapy for cirrhotic sodium retention was introduced by Murray Epstein of Miami who found that immersion in water at 34°C up to the neck in a seated position (in a 4 ft deep bath) likewise causes a sodium diuresis apparently by increasing central plasma volume: the water pressure compresses the legs and body so increasing central venous volume and causing a sodium diuresis. I have observed a similar response in nephrotics.

Question In renal failure would you use aldactone (spironolactone)?

Answer 1. Yes. Go on to **2.68**.
         2. Go on to **2.70**.

2.70 Your answer—no. Aldactone should not be given in renal failure.
        You are correct. If a patient who is not in renal failure is resistant to diuretics we can do two things. 1. Increase the dose of Lasix by doubling it daily until there is a response or a dose of 1—2 g is needed. Remember that i.v. Lasix is more effective than oral Lasix because Lasix acts on the tubules from the luminal side i.e. it has to be in a high enough concentration *inside* the lumen, and this is aided by the Lasix being given i.v.—i.v. injection rapidly causes higher blood levels after i.v. injection than the same dose given by mouth. If more than 100 mg is given per hour temporary buzzing and deafness may be complained of so that it is wisest to give it as an intravenous infusion in obstinate cases—say 500 mg over 5 hours. If even high dose Lasix fails then oedema can be removed by haemofiltration i.e. passing the blood through an artificial kidney, on which a negative transmembrane pressure is applied by a vacuum pump,

so ultrafiltering the plasma. This way 2 or 3 litres of ECF can be safely removed per hour without hypotension. To mitigate the difficulties of a low sodium diet, potassium and ammonium cycle ion-exchange renins were once given to bind sodium. These have fallen into disfavour because they need a close watch on the electrolytes and may precipitate hepatic coma in cirrhotics. Similarly oral 70 per cent sorbitol given in 40 ml doses every 20 minutes can induce a diarrhoea containing about 100 mEq of sodium and 20 to 30 mEq of potassium per litre. It is however an unpleasant way of getting rid of ECF and quite inferior to haemofiltration or dialysis, but may be needed if artificial kidneys are not available. Southey's tubes (the old and out dated method of draining oedema by inserting little silver tubes into the oedematous legs subcutaneously and allowing the oedema fluid to drain through rubber tubes into a bottle), are mentioned only in case you may be asked about them by some 'museum piece' who used them before modern efficient therapy became available with powerful diuretics. A recently reintroduced thiazide metolazone is a very powerful diuretic and may work when Lasix does not. It is always worth a trial before haemo-filtration.

Now look carefully at the 3 statements below:

Statement 1. Exchangeable sodium is lower than Total Body Sodium.
Statement 2. Hypernatraemia is usually due to sodium excess.
Statement 3. Hyponatraemia occurs commonly in cirrhosis of the liver.

Now choose the answers which are in your opinion correct.

1. Statement 1 is true, 2 and 3 false. Go on to **2.41**.
2. Statement 2 is true, 1 and 3 false. Go on to **2.43**.
3. Statement 3 is true, 1 and 2 false. Go on to **2.46**.
4. All statements are true. Go on to **2.48**.
5. Statement 1 is false, 2 and 3 true. Go on to **2.50**.
6. Statement 2 is false, 1 and 3 true. Go on to **2.52**.
7. Statement 3 is false, 2 and 3 true. Go on to **2.53**.
8. All statements are false. Go on to **2.54**.

2.71   Your answer—3 kg. No. You are guessing. Read **2.66** again.

Time for this chapter: $1\frac{1}{2}$ hours.

Chapter 3
Potassium

3.1   Potassium is the major intracellular cation, but is also found in low but critical concentration in the extracellular fluid. Its concentration in the plasma varies from 3.4 to 5.6 mEq/ litre in health although it must be remembered that the plasma levels of potassium do *not* reflect the total intracellular potassium content. It is possible to get high plasma K figures with depleted total body K stores and low plasma K concentrations with low total body K stores. At present it appears that about 2/3 of intra-cellular K is bound; this is revealed by micro-electrodes inserted into the cell and having specific sensitivity for K ion. The potassium content in the body is about 45 $\pm$ 4 mEq/kg in men and about 37 $\pm$ 3 mEq/kg in women, as measured by exchangeable potassium using ^{42}K. Total body potassium stores, like sodium stores, are measurable directly only in the cadaver, with ashing of the body and dissolving of the ash in mineral acid. Following this labourious procedure, it is possible to obtain accurate figures for total body potassium in the entire cadaver, but it obviously is a totally impractical method for clinical use, as well as a particularly abhorrent method for acquiring data. For clinical use there are two excellent methods. Both are based on radioactivity measurements: (1) ^{40}K measurement. ^{40}K is a naturally occurring isotope of potassium which is found throughout nature and is present as a fixed percentage of stable non-radioactive potassium. ^{40}K is weakly radioactive and can be readily measured in a whole body counter which is well shielded from external radiation—even the brick walls of a building contain enough ^{40}K to interfere with the whole body counter's ^{40}K measurement. The proportion of ^{40}K to stable K is fixed, and knowing the ^{40}K content it is a simple matter to calculate the amount of stable K. The results of measurements of total body potassium using ^{40}K in the whole body counter are in good agreement with those obtained by direct physical measurement in the whole cadaver.

Now answer the question:

Question ^{40}K is:

Answer 1. Non-radioactive. Go on to **3.2**.
2. Radioactive and naturally occurring. Go on to **3.3**.
3. Radioactive and made in an atomic pile. Go on to **3.5**.

3.2 Your answer—^{40}K is non-radioactive.

You are wrong. You have not been concentrating while reading **3.1**. Go back and read **3.1** again. Then answer the question. Incidentally you must put away all distractions; your answer indicates that you are not paying attention to the work. Switch off all TVs, or radios, casettes or phonographs in the room—if you cannot stop the distractions, stop learning until you can do so without them. Do not fool yourself, ever.

3.3 Your answer—It is radioactive and naturally occurring.

You are correct. Let us continue with how to measure total K in the body *in vivo*. The ^{42}K method is similar to the ^{24}Na and ^{22}Na methods you have already read about in Chapter 2. Exchangeable potassium or K_E is determined by giving a known amount of ^{42}K by mouth (half life 12.5 hours) and collecting the urine for 24 hours. After this period of equilibration the concentration of ^{42}K and stable potassium are determined in the plasma or a fresh sample of urine. The calculation is done as follows, after correction of the counts for the short half life ^{42}K isotope:

Dose of isotope given	25,000 cpm
Loss of isotope in the urine in 24 hours	4,000 cpm
Total amount ^{42}K retained	21,000 cpm

After 24 hr. Concentration of stable K in plasma = 4.5 mEq/l
After 24 hr. Concentration of ^{42}K in plasma = 31.5 cp/l

Specific activity of plasma $=\dfrac{31.5}{4.5}$ = 7 cpm/mEq

Exchangeable potassium (K_E) $= \dfrac{21,000}{7}$

$= 3,000$ mEq

Measurements of K_E are about 15 per cent less than measurements of total body potassium using ^{40}K, presumably due to incompleteness of penetration of ^{42}K into the deeper layers of bone in the 24 hour period of equilibration. The distribution of potassium is principally in the cells. Thus out of a total of 3,800 mEq of potassium in the body there are only 12 mEq in the plasma. The majority of the potassium, 2730 mEq, is found in the skeletal muscle; look at Table 3.3

"Organ"	mEqK
Muscle (Skeletal)	2730
Skin	360
Red blood cells	252
Bone	218
Brain	150
Liver	135
Heart	24
Kidneys	18

This is strikingly different from sodium, where out of a total of 5000 mEq in the entire body 1600 mEq are found in skin and 1600 mEq in bone and 363 mEq in the plasma. Of course sodium is the principal *extracellular* cation and potassium is the major *intracellular* cation. Also note that very little K is found in skin and bone, whereas much sodium is found in both these sites. Read this paragraph again, please, and study Table 3.3.
    Now answer the question:

Question Out of a total of 3800 mEq of potassium in the body, 2730 mEq are found in what tissue?

Answer 1. Plasma. Go on to **3.4**.
    2. Skeletal muscle. Go on to **3.7**.
    3. Bone. Go on to **3.9**.

3.4   Your answer—2730 mEq of K are found in the plasma.

No. You are a bad guesser and a lazy one at that. In the plasma there are 4 mEq/litre, and the plasma volume is 2.5 to 3 litres i.e. there are < 12 mEq in the plasma. Go back and read **3.3** again.

3.5   Your answer—it is radioactive and made in an atomic pile.
    You are guessing. ^{40}K is radioactive, but it is a natural isotope found throughout nature. The answer you choose indicates you do not know the material in **3.1**. Read **3.1** again, this time carefully and without distractions. If you can, sit by yourself in a quiet comfortable room away from other people. If you can't then stop 'learning' until you can get circumstances which permit you to learn rather than day-dream.

3.6   Your answer—There is no K in chips (french fries).

You are wrong and have not read **3.7** carefully. Go and read it again. Concentrate on what you are reading this time.

3.7   Your answer—2730 mEq of K out of a total of 3800 mEq are found in skeletal muscle.

You are correct. ^{42}K has a particularly short life of just over 12 hours. If one measures K_E with equilibration periods of 48 and 72 hours there is a progressive increase in K_E decreasing the gap between K_E and ^{40}K total body potassium results, but the measurements get less accurate because of the short half life of ^{42}K (6 half lives have decayed by 72 hours so the accuracy of the count may be low). In the normal diet potassium intake is from about 60 mEq to 200 mEq a day depending on the intake of meat and fruit. Raisins, sultanas, dried apricots and dried peaches contain much potassium—in the region of 25 mEq/100 g, whereas in cooked meats there is about 8 mEq/100 g. Bear in mind that the content of potassium in the raw food can be considerably reduced by the method of cooking. Potatoes are particularly full of potassium. There are 100 mEq of K in 100 g of chips (french fries); about 75 mEq of K in 100 g of roast potatoes; and 30 mEq of K in 100 g of boiled potatoes. Thus boiling the potatoes in water which is then poured away and replaced by fresh water reduces the potassium content of the final product considerably, as Shaldon pointed out. A diet free of potassium can be readily achieved by giving milk which has been passed through an ion exchange resin in the sodium cycle as developed by Black and Milne in their classic potassium depletion experiment. Otherwise it is quite difficult to achieve a K free diet.

Now answer the question:

Question What is the amount of potassium in 100 g of chips (french fries)?

Answer 1. There is no potassium in them. Go on to **3.6**.
2. 100 mEq of K. Go on to **3.8**.
3. 10 mEq of K. Go on to **3.10**.

3.8   Your answer—100 mEq of K/100 g of chips (french fries).

Good. The physiological control of potassium balance is far less effic-ient than that of sodium. The urine in a normal person contains potassium in quantities of 10 to 20 mEq/day even when a potassium-free diet is taken i.e. a persistent urinary potassium leak is normal. Thus potassium deficiency is easy to achieve, just by having a K free intake. In contrast when a sodium-free diet is given the urine becomes virtually sodium-free i.e. contains 1 to 2 mEq/day indicating a remarkably efficient physiological mechanism for sodium conservation. In a person on a normal diet the urine contains about 100 mEq/day, and thus is dependent on the potassium intake, level of plasma potassium, acid-base balance, diuretics, aldosterone and corticosteroids. Before discussing these factors in detail it is worthwhile to recall some of the details of the normal renal handling of potassium. Potassium circulates in the plasma in free state i.e. not bound to protein. It is therefore freely filtered at the glomerulus so that in normal man about 500 μEq/min are filtered at a plasma K level of 4 mEq/ litre and a GFR of 120 ml/min. Do the calculations yourself thus, 4 mEq/ litre = 4 μEq/ml. Each minute 120 ml of plasma are filtered containing 120 $\times$ 4 μEq of K = 480 μEq/min.

85 per cent of filtered potassium is reabsorbed in the renal tubules, 15 per cent being excreted in the urine. There is evidence that most if not all the filtered potassium is reabsorbed proximally and that which appears in the urine is due to distal secretion in the distal tubule and collecting ducts. In renal failure the amount of potassium secreted increases until the clearance of potassium exceeds that of inulin i.e., there is overall tubular secretion of potassium in renal failure, potassium clearance approaching up to two to three times the glomerular filtration rate.

Now answer the question:

Question How much tubular reabsorption of filtered potassium is found in a healthy man?

Answer 1. 10 per cent. Go on to **3.11**.

           2. 85 per cent. Go on to **3.15**.

3.9 Your answer—2730 mEq of K are found in bone.

Your answer is a guess, and it is wrong. Bone has only a little K in its crystal lattice. You are guessing. Read **3.3** again.

3.10 Your answer—10 mEq K/100 g chips.

No. You have not remembered **3.7** adequately. Read it again. You have a ten fold error.

3.11 Your answer—10 per cent of filtered K is reabsorbed.

You have not concentrated. Most of the filtered K is reabsorbed, otherwise the body would be depleted of potassium in a few days. Go back and read **3.8** more carefully. And this time do not day-dream.

3.12   Your answer—hyperkalaemia.

You really are not concentrating. Had you read **3.15** with any care you would have learned that hyperkalaemia has quite characteristic signs on an ECG. You must be distracted. Shut the book and come back to **3.8** when you can concentrate without any difficulty.

3.13   Your answer—15 per cent of filtered K is reabsorbed.

No, you have not read **3.8** carefully. 85 per cent of filtered K is re-absorbed and if this were not so you would need to take a huge K intake to remain alive—say 400 mEq/day. Read **3.8** again carefully.

3.14   Your answer—The ECG shows changes of hypokalaemia. You have made the correct choice.

Good. What are the factors affecting the plasma potassium level? Firstly there is the state of repletion or depletion of the potassium stores of the body. It should be stressed that although generally hypokalaemia is associated with potassium depletion and hyperkalaemia associated most frequently with normal or increased body stores, this is by no means a hard and fast rule. There are rapid changes in plasma potassium concentration which can give hyperkalaemia in the presence of depleted body reserves; similarly hypokalaemia may be found despite normal body stores of potassium.

The causes of hyperkalaemia are given in Table 3.14. Learn it. In any case where the cause of hyperkalaemia is not immediately apparent, exclude haemolysis by examining the colour of the plasma before it is sent to the laboratory and do *not* squirt the blood through a needle into the tube. If haemolysis is not present, then an excessively high platelet count may be responsible—in this case the high K is due to liberation of K from the platelets on clotting of the blood. Thus *serum* has a high K concentration and *plasma* has a normal K concentration. What can cause very rapid changes in plasma K levels? Two frequent examples are changes in plasma pH—e.g. hyperventilation (due to hysteria or over-ventilation on a respirator) with resultant respiratory alkalosis i.e. a rise in plasma pH; or hypoventilation as a result of barbiturate or similar sedative overdosage causing respiratory depression and a fall in plasma pH. A rough guide to the magnitude of the change is *a fall in plasma pH of 0.1 unit causes a rise in plasma K level of 1 mEq/l.* This is a rough and ready guide indicating how a rapid change in plasma K can be brought about without change in intracellular potassium reserves. If you are faced with a patient with an abnormal plasma K, make sure you have

Table 3.14.   Hyperkalaemia causes (modified from Gabow)

---

1. *Pseudohyperkalaemia*
   Tourniquet method of drawing blood
   Haemolysis of drawn blood
   Increased WBC or platelet count
2. *True Hyperkalaemia*
   (a) Redistribution
        Acidosis
        Hyperkalaemic familial periodic paralysis
   (b) Decreased excretion
        Chronic or acute renal failure
        Potassium-sparing diuretics
        Deficiency of adrenal steroids
           Addison's disease
           Hyporeninemic hypoaldosteronism (Type IV RTA)
   (c) Increased production
        Haemolysis
        Muscle trauma, Rhabdomyolysis
   (d) Increased Intake
           Potassium citrate, Fruit.

Learn this list. Keep writing it out with the book closed until you know it.

plasma pH figures to help your interpretation and influence your treatment. Time after time I have to drum this into aspiring nephrologists who
want to make life and death therapeutic decisions without sufficient data.
So don't be lazy. Get the data.

If glucose is infused with insulin there is a rapid fall in plasma K
level due to K entering the cells when there is glycogen synthesis. This
fall in plasma K induced by glucose and insulin infusion is of importance
in the treatment of hyperkalaemia.

Now answer the question.

Question What level of serum potassium would you expect if a man who
had originally a plasma arterial pH of 7.31 and a serum potassium of
5.0 mEq/l and suddenly developed airways obstruction and a fall in
arterial pH to 7.21?

Answer 1. Serum (K) of 4 mEq/l. Go on to **3.16**.
2. Serum (K) of 2 mEq/l. Go on to **3.18**.
3. Serum (K) of 6 mEq/l. Go on to **3.20**.

3.15   Your answer—about 85 per cent is reabsorbed.

Good. The concentration of potassium in the plasma in normal health is found to be between 3.4 and 5.6 mEq/l. There is remarkably little room for safety if the plasma level falls or rises. If the plasma level of K falls to 2.0 mEq/l or below there is interference with normal muscular function, both cardiac and skeletal. This is hardly surprising, in view of the major role that potassium has in the genesis of the normal muscle membrane potential, which is largely a function of the ratio of the concentrations of intracellular potassium and extracellular potassium i.e. K concentration on either side of the membranes i.e. (K int)/(K ext). When the muscle contracts, the action potential is associated with the ejection of a small amount of intracellular potassium. Thus because a fall in plasma potassium is accompanied by a fall in the extracellular fluid potassium concentration, the ratio (K int)/(K ext) rises, the membrane potential rises and the muscle is more irritable. If intracellular K is depleted, and this is usually the case in the condition of severe hypokalaemia, then the membrane potential falls and the muscle may become less irritable. In advanced cases of intracellular K depletion the entire contractile mechanism may be seriously impaired. Let us look at the cardiac changes:

Cardiac changes: Low external concentrations of potassium reduce the amount of potassium going back into the cell i.e. reduce repolarization, so that there is a depression of the ST segment and a lowering of the height of the T wave on the ECG and a prominent U wave which may be biphasic. Look at Fig. 3.15a. The reverse occurs with a high ECF potassium concentration when there is an *increase* in repolarization so that there is an elevation of the ST segment with high peaked T waves. This is a characteristic sign of hyperkalaemia. Look at Fig. 3.15b. AV conduction is depressed in the presence of hypokalaemia. In addition in patients receiving digitalis glycosides, potassium depletion causes an increase in cardiac arrhythmias including nodal tachycardia, paroxysmal atrial tachycardia with atrio-ventricular block, ventricular extrasystoles, and finally ventricular fibrillation.

Skeletal muscle changes in hypokalaemia: Weakness of skeletal muscles starts in the limbs peripherally and spreads centrally, eventually to involve the respiratory muscles with respiratory failure.

Paralytic ileus may occur with severe hypokalaemia. *Tetany.* Potassium depletion, predominantly intracellular, is responsible for the production of tetany manifested initally as paraesthesiae in the extremities and progressing to carpopedal spasm and even convulsions.

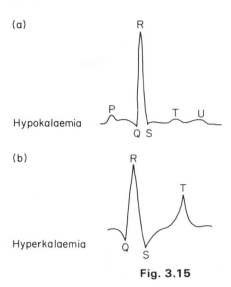

Fig. 3.15

Renal changes: In hypokalaemia there is an inability to concentrate the urine, associated with a proximal tubular vacuolation histologically. The urine hypo-osmolality of hypokalaemia may be reversed by indomethacin administration indicating that the inability to concentrate the urine is prostaglandin mediated.

In Hyperkalaemia there are cardiac and skeletal muscle effects. The cardiac effects are (I) *indirect*, on the conduction mechanism with a reduced AV conduction time and (II) *direct* effect on the myocardium producing either ventricular arrest or ventricular fibrillation. Skeletal musculature becomes paralysed in hyperkalaemia as in hypokalaemia, the paralysis moving centripetally from the limbs and leading finally to respiratory arrest. Now look at the ECG. What does it indicate?

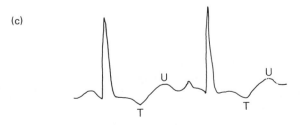

Fig. 3.15

Answer 1. Hypokalaemia. Go on to **3.12**.
           2. Hypokalaemia. Go on to **3.14**.

3.16 Your answer—a serum K of 4 mEq/l.
     If you had read **3.14** with care you would have seen that for each fall of plasma pH of 0.1 units, the K rises by 1 mEq/l. You should read **3.14** again, then answer the question correctly.

3.17 Your answer—increased entry of potassium into the cells.
     No. You are guessing with little thought. Go back and read **3.20** with more care. If you cannot, then stop reading. This is not a novel, nor can you speed read through it. Read every word carefully.

3.18 Your answer—a serum K of 2 mEq/l.
     You are guessing. Read **3.14** again. If you cannot concentrate, do not waste your time. Try and get rid of distractive interferences. If you are unable to do this, take a break, then go back to **3.14** when circumstances are more favourable.

3.19 Your answer—increased loss of potassium is due to cellular breakdown.
     You are correct. The causes of K depletion are given in Table 3.19. Hypokalaemia is found in patients who are suffering from hyperaldosteronism, either primary (which is rare) and most frequently due to adenoma of the adrenal cortex, or secondary, which is most commonly due to the administration of diuretics, nephrotic syndrome, renal artery stenosis, hypoproteinaemia of any cause and also uraemia. The cause of this hypokalaemia is the continual loss of potassium caused by stimulation of potassium secretion by aldosterone in the distal sites of potassium secretion by aldosterone in the distal sites of potassium secretion in the distal tubules and in the collecting ducts. Clinically hypokalaemia is not accompanied by any symptoms until the plasma K level has fallen to the vicinity of 2.0 mEq/l (i.e. a loss of 200–300 mEq of K has occurred) when there may be interference with the ability to produce a concentrated urine. This is manifested clinically by nocturia and polyuria, with elaboration of a hypotonic urine whose osmolality remains below that of plasma—despite the administration of exogenous vasopressin i.e. a form of *nephrogenic diabetes insipidus*. Histologically there is vacuolation of the proximal

Table 3.19.   Causes of potassium deficiency
(after Schrier)

Apparent Potassium Deficit
  Alkalosis
  Familial hypokalaemic periodic paralysis
True Potassium Deficit
  Poor Dietary Intake
    Alcoholism
    Anorexia nervosa
    Clay ingestion
  Gastro-intestinal Loss
    Pyloric stenosis
    Diarrhoea
    Laxative abuse
    Ureterosigmoidostomy
    Ileal loop bladder
    Villous adenoma
  Urinary Loss
    Diuretic therapy
    Excessive mineralocorticoid effect
      Primary and secondary hyperaldosteronism
      Cushing's syndrome
      Licorice abuse
      Bartter's syndrome
    Renal tubular acidosis
      Osmotic diuretic
      Chronic interstitial nephritis

Learn this Table, then write it out 5 times with the book closed.

and collecting tubules, and the condition of hypokalaemic nephropathy is
accompanied by pyelonephritis more frequently than could be accounted
for by chance alone. In Bartter's syndrome there is potassium loss in the
urine leading to severe K store depletion and low plasma, K levels, with
high plasma angiotension levels but without hypertension. The juxta-
glomerular apparatus is hypertrophied on renal biopsy. The cause is
unknown, but because it partially responds to the administration of
indomethacin, a prostaglandin synthetase inhibitor, it seems to be caused
by an excess of prostaglandins of unknown aetiology. Cushing's syndrome
due to glucocorticoid excess caused by adrenal cortical hyperplasia or

tumour, or secondary to extra adrenal neoplasm, such as carcinoma of the bronchus, may be associated with hypokalaemia, frequently more severe in the latter group of extra-adrenal corticosteroid synthesis. Primary renal disease may lead to K loss: a striking cause is potassium losing nephritis, usually a rare complication of pyelonephritis. Renal tubular disease such as Fanconi syndrome and distal renal tubular acidosis may be responsible for massive total body K depletion with severe hypokalaemia necessitating vigorous potassium repletion. Remember, *proximal renal tubular acidosis (RTA) does not regularly produce K depletion—but distal RTA does produce K depletion regularly.*

Question A man is found to be suffering from severe hypokalaemia (serum K level 1.8 mEq/l), without hypertension but with high plasma renin activity, and on renal biopsy has hypertrophied juxta-glomerula apparatus. To what drug will the hypokalaemia respond?

Answer 1. Indomethacin. Go on to **3.21**.
2. Cortisone. Go on to **3.23**.
3. Potassium chloride. Go on to **3.25**.

3.20 Your answer—a serum K of 6 mEq/l.
Good. You are correct. In anabolic states, when protein is laid down, K enters the cells in a ratio of 2.7 mEq of potassium for every gram of nitrogen. Remember this figure *2.7 mEq K per g of Nitrogen*. Thus if a patient is in positive nitrogen balance, such as when he is recovering from an operation after the initial catabolic state, say we find he has a positive nitrogen balance of 5 g/day. Now because 6.25 g of protein contains 1 g of nitrogen, then he is laying down 5 × 6.25 g of protein a day = 31.25 g of protein. We would expect that he would also be in positive balance for potassium of 5 × 2.7 = 13.5 mEq per day, just taking his protein anabolism only into account. Similarly in a growing child a positive nitrogen balance is accompanied by a positive potassium balance. In catabolic patients i.e. those who are breaking down their body tissues at a greater rate than they are building them up, there is a negative *nitrogen* balance accompanied by a negative *potassium* balance. Read this last sentence again. Catabolic states occur in infections, starvation, trauma (including surgical operations) and burns. In catabolic states there will be a loss of potassium from the cells paralleling the nitrogen loss. If there is a degree of renal failure the cellular loss of potassium in catabolic states may cause a rise in plasma potassium levels, resulting in hyperkalaemia, this being exacerbated by the frequently accompanying metabolic uraemic acidosis.

Hyperkalaemia is a frequent cause of death in patients with severe catabolic states and renal failure such as after trauma or burns. Hyperkalaemia may also be found in hypoaldosteronism, where the plasma aldosterone is very low, and plasma renin concentration is high. In hyporeninic hypoaldosteronism, hyperkalaemia is found with a low plasma renin and a low plasma aldosterone level.

Question In hypercatabolic renal failure the serum potassium level rises more rapidly than in non-hypercatabolic states. Why?

Answer 1. Increased entry of potassium into the cell. Go on to **3.17**.
2. Increased loss of potassium from cells due to cellular breakdown. Go on to **3.19**.

3.21 Your answer—Indomethacin.

You are correct. Gastro-intestinal disease is a common cause of potassium depletion. Severe diarrhoea of any origin may cause massive potassium loss in the faeces, and in addition there may be interference with the absorption of potassium from the small intestine, or potassium in food may not reach the small intestine due to vomiting or anorexia. Thus potassium depletion may occur in steatorrhoea of any cause, e.g. Crohn's disease, ulcerative colitis; and Ellison–Zollinger syndrome. The diarrhoea of purgation due to laxative abuse is noteworthy as causing severe hypokalaemia on occasion. Another cause is a potassium secreting papilloma of the rectum and colon. Pyloric stenosis accompanied by copious vomiting is a well documented cause of potassium depletion as well as sodium depletion. It is essential in treating this condition not to forget to replace the potassium depleted reserves *before* operation to prevent cardiac arrhythmia occurring during the subsequent operation. One of the most frequent and dangerous types of potassium depletion occurs in the post-operative surgical patient with ileus, who is on a 'suck and drip regimen' in whom potassium-containing fluid is being continuously drained from the small intestine but in whom inadequate restitution of the potassium is being made, due to lack of measurement of all the K lost including the inevitable urinary loss. Often the surgical case of this type has multiple abdominal drains and so many complicated facets that the surgeon may simply be so distracted as to forget adequate replacement of potassium. A similar problem may be found in any patient dependent on i.v. fluids: the potassium loss may be compounded by a loss of magnesium and phosphate pari-passu.

Now answer the question:

Question A patient is admitted to hospital in a sodium depleted state with a low blood pressure due to pyloric stenosis. Before operation he should have his ECF volume repleted with the i.v. administration of sodium chloride and another cation. Which cation?

Answer 1. He needs calcium. Go on to **3.22**.
2. He needs magnesium. Go on to **3.24**.
3. He needs phosphate. Go on to **3.26**.
4. He needs potassium. Go on to **3.28**.

3.22 Your answer—he needs calcium.
You are wrong. No sense in guessing. Now read **3.21** with greater care. This time concentrate.

3.23 Your answer—cortisone.
No. You are guessing. Go and read **3.19** with more concentration. Then choose the correct answer.

3.24 Your answer—he needs magnesium.
You are partially correct but confusing drip and suction with pyloric stenosis. Read **3.21** again, but pay attention this time.

3.25 Your answer—potassium chloride.
That is a good guess but unfortunately it will not cure Bartter's syndrome. Go back and read about it again in **3.19**.

3.26 Your answer—he needs phosphate.
Some patients do become phosphate depleted but this is more frequent with a drip and suction regime, and phosphate should not be your choice because it is not a cation but an anion. Read **3.21** again, carefully this time.

3.27 Your answer—100 per cent.
You are wrong. No need to guess. It is simpler to read **3.28** carefully, than waste your time guessing.

3.28 Your answer—he needs potassium.
Good. In familial periodic paralysis there is one group of patients in which the muscular paralysis is related to the sudden appearance of hypokalaemia caused by the redistribution of K in the body with a shift from ECF to ICF. It is treated/or prevented by oral K salts. Do not forget

that in *severe hypokalaemia of any aetiology acute rhabdomyolysis may occur*, with severe paralysis, muscle soreness, myoglobinaemia and myoglobinuria and raised CPK levels. What is the level of K depletion that is associated with symptoms? Black suggested that at least 200 mEq must be lost (or 10 per cent of the body K stores) before any symptoms occur. In experimental studies of Fourman 10–30 per cent depletion of total body K was associated with muscle weakness, intolerance to cold, thirst, apathy, tetany, oedema: and U waves on the ECG were seen. Because there was also sodium depletion and acidosis, correction of these removed some of the symptoms. If more than 30 per cent of total body potassium is depleted, the patient develops renal diabetes insipidus with polyuria, inability to gain weight post-operatively, ileus and finally muscular paralysis. There is a rise in plasma pH, associated with an intracellular increase in hydrogen ion with loss of this hydrogen ion from the ECF. The magnitude of the hydrogen ion entry into the cells, if it occurs, is however not of sufficient magnitude to explain the acidosis fully. Severe hypokalaemia blocks the secretion of aldosterone, so there is a high renin and low aldosterone level and a urine rich in chloride and sodium.

Now answer the question:

Question How much of the body potassium needs to be lost before symptoms occur?

Answer 1. 100 per cent. Go on to **3.27**.
2. 10–30 per cent. Go on to **3.29**.
3. 1 per cent. Go on to **3.31**.

3.29   Your answer—10–30 per cent.
You are correct. Now let us look at:

The treatment of hypokalaemia and potassium depletion. When the plasma K levels falls below 3.4 mEq/litre, total body potassium is frequently depleted and needs replenishing. It is wise at this stage to measure the 24 hour urine K output. If K output is more than 50 mEq with a plasma K of less than 3.5 mEq/litre then a renal K wasting disorder is present. If the K excretion is less than 50 mEq/day a gastro-intestinal disorder is probably present. If the K level is 2.5 mEq/litre or less intravenous replenishment should be made with KCl at a rate of 10 mEq/hour with monitoring of plasma K levels every 2 hours and continuous monitoring of the ECG in an intensive care unit. It is wise to err on the side of conservatism when considering potassium replenishment because too energetic i.v., therapy may result in fatal hyperkalaemia with cardiac arrest, despite a total body K of less than normal levels. In severe K depletion of chronic type oral replenishment using Mist Pot. Cit. (potassium citrate 30 g/100 ml) in which 15 ml contains 28 mEq of potassium so give 15 ml 3 times a day = 84 mEq/day. Diuretic potassium depletion may require the addition of chloride in large quantities (as ammonium chloride) before potassium is adequately retained and the hypokalaemic alkalosis cured by means of expanding to normal the contracted ECF volume. Remember that in hypokalaemia there is an extracellular alkalosis, hydrogen ions having left the ECF and entered the cells replacing lost ICF potassium causing an intracellular acidosis. Thus in hypokalaemia there is a urine produced with a high ammonia concentration. This highly acid urine excretion exacerbates the hypokalaemic alkalosis.

Potassium depletion causes a reduction in aldosterone production so that severe hypokalaemia is often associated with low levels of plasma aldosterone, renin levels remaining high. Consequently, sodium and chloride excretion are enhanced in many patients with hypokalaemia as a result of the fall in plasma aldosterone levels and also as a result of intracellular acidosis in the renal tubular cells.

In the therapy of diabetic ketosis potassium levels may fall strikingly as glucose re-enters the cells under the influence of insulin, causing hypokalaemia. Often there is an antecedent massive reduction in total body potassium especially if the acidosis is of several weeks' standing and is associated with an osmotic glucose diuresis and the urinary loss of β-hydroxybutyrate. In this case potassium has to be supplied intravenously to restore plasma K levels to normal or at least safe levels.

Oral KCl tablets or liquids are known to be occasionally associated with ulceration of the small intestine with ulcers complicated by perforation and stenosis. This has been shown to occur if the local potassium concentration exceeds 7 mEq/1. For this purpose slow release K tablets such as slow K were designed with the KCl held inside a resinous base so that its dissolution is particularly slow, but even these in very rare instances have been associated with small bowel ulceration. It is best to replenish K loss, say chronic loss due to diuretics, with potato chips (french fries) or dried fruit. In diarrhoea, chips are often edible, but obviously dried figs and prunes should be eschewed to prevent further exacerbation of diarrhoea. It is easier and more pleasant to replace 100 mEq of K with a few ounces of chips or dried apricots than all the slow release or other K tablets, and at least as effective; and considerably cheaper into the bargain. Remember that chips *do not* cause small intestinal ulceration nor do dried fruits! So make your choice knowing food K content rather than the latest advertisement for potassium salts appearing in the Journals. Obviously if the patient is a laxative addict there must be a vigorous attempt to prevent them getting the laxatives and to give the patient appropriate psychological support during this weaning process, as well as getting at the root of the problem to prevent relapse or worse if the laxative is not replaced with some alternative psychological crutch. In the patient suffering from a potassium secreting papilloma of the large bowel it is wise to attempt to replete potassium to make anaesthesia safe, but then to lose no time in extirpating the tumour.

Now answer the question.

Question A man has been given Lasix for 2 years, 40 mg a day. He has a plasma potassium level of 2.5 mEq/litre, and a plasma pH of 7.5 and he has 10 mEq of potassium in the urine. He has been treated with 50 mEq of potassium citrate, and this resulted in a marginal rise of potassium to 2.7 mEq/l. What additional therapy would you give with potassium ion to effect a cure of hypokalaemic alkalosis?

Answer 1. Bicarbonate as $NaHCO_3$. Go on to **3.30**.
2. Ammonium chloride. Go on to **3.32**.
3. Potassium hydroxide. Go on to **3.34**.

3.30 Your answer—give bicarbonate.
No. Your mind wandered when you were reading **3.29**. Read it again.

3.31 Your answer—1 per cent. You are guessing.
Go back and read **3.28** again. Concentrate this time. Turn off your radio, T.V., records or tapes. Then try to read **3.28** again.

3.32 Your answer—ammonium chloride.
You are correct.

The treatment of hyperkalaemia is of primary importance; it is a medical emergency, and the principles of treatment of this common complication of renal failure should be *understood* fully in addition to being learned.

The main principles are: Speed and Safety.

1. Start at once. Get an *ECG lead II* to confirm the high peaked T waves. Do *not* wait for laboratory confirmation. The order is important. Then go on to the following steps:

Injection i.v. of calcium ion which directly antagonizes the effect of potassium on the myocardium and so protects the heart from fatal arrhythmias. This is of immediate importance and in practice *20 ml of 10 per cent calcium gluconate* is given i.v. over five minutes. This contains about 180 mg of elemental calcium (90 mg for *10* ml of 10 per cent calcium gluconate). Which is it wiser to give—calcium gluconate or chloride, and how much? The answer is as follows: calcium gluconate is not likely to cause tissue necrosis if it gets outside the veins. Similarly it is not acidic, whereas $CaCl_2$ is. However the amount of elemental calcium in 10 ml of 10 per cent calcium chloride is 360 mg and in the same volume and concentration of calcium gluconate it is 90 mg. Assuming that we want to elevate the ionized calcium level by at least one mg per 100 ml, to counteract the myocardial effects of hyperkalaemia in some way, and that there are 15 litres of ECF in which the calcium given will rapidly distribute, then 10 ml of 10 per cent $CaCl_2$ will contribute $360/15,000 \times 100$ mg/ 100 ml of $Ca^{2+} = 2.4$ mg/100 ml. On the other hand calcium gluconate in the same volume and strength will contribute $90/15,000 \times 100$ mg of ionized calcium/100 ml $= 0.6$ mg/100 ml. It is therefore obvious that the choice should be either *20* ml of 10 per cent calcium gluconate or 10 ml of calcium chloride given slowly. If there is serious hypocalcaemia in absolute terms then calcium chloride is better. After this the patient can be given sodium bicarbonate intravenously which will not only elevate the plasma pH but also drive potassium back into the cell. If you have a patient with poor veins inject the solutions slowly into an intravenous infusion line after you have made sure that it is not going into the paravenous tissues. The vein can be kept open with 0.9l saline infusion.

2. Correct acidosis. This is the *second* step, because correction of an acidosis in the presence of a low plasma calcium will reduce plasma ionized calcium even further and may cause tetanic convulsions with the possibility of fractures of the diseased bones in renal disease. Fracture of the femur can be caused in patients with chronic renal disease by some enthusiastic physician treating with sodium bicarbonate an asymptomatic or chronic acidosis revealed by acid base studies. PRIMUM NON NOCERE—'first do not harm'. Always give calcium i.v. first, then sodium bicarbonate in a dose of 100 mEq over 5 minutes, and do not give any more until plasma K and plasma pH have been checked 15−30 minutes after the last dose of bicarbonate. Giving calcium first and then $NaHCO_3$ will prevent a dangerous fall of ionized calcium and tetanic convulsions. Then go on to give more bicarbonate if the plasma calcium is normal. The total amount of $NaHCO_3$ to be given has to be calculated assuming a volume of distribution of 2/3 body weight. *But give it in small doses repeatedly with repeated plasma pH and PCO_2 measurements.* Use this biochemical and ECG servo mechanism and you will save lives, not kill people.

3. Give insulin 20 u (soluble) **with 50 g of glucose** i.v. This causes potassium to go into the cells with glycogen synthesis, but this causes only a *temporary* fall of plasma K levels: after a few hours the plasma K levels rise again, probably by leaking out from the cells. It is known that glucose alone will cause a fall in K, but it is safer to give i.v. insulin and *ensure* the entry of K into the liver.

4. Give ion exchange resins. There are two common forms of cation exchange resin in use—the first being Kay-exalate (Resonium A) a sodium containing form of polystyrene sulphonate. This is an efficient ion exchange resin and exchanges its Na^+ for other ions in the intestine *including* K^+. It works in a few hours, but gives the patient sodium ion in exchange. This oral dose of 60 g per day causes an average of 120 mEq of sodium to be absorbed and 60 mEq of K (1 mEq K per g of resin) to be removed. The sodium absorption may, in a few days, cause serious problems for the patient including massive ECF expansion with attendant right heart failure, hypertension, left heart failure and fits. Because of this danger in the renal failure patient it is advisable not to use Kay-exalate unless the patient is *sodium depleted.* The second resin which I introduced instead of Kay-exalate is the calcium cycle form Zeocarb 225. This works slightly less efficiently than the sodium cycle resin in removing potassium, but exchanges potassium ion for calcium ion the latter being absorbed with difficulty in renal failure. Nevertheless daily plasma calcium levels should be measured to detect the rare case of hypercalcaemia as a result of calcium absorption and thus to reduce the dose. Calcium resin is not available in the U.S.A., but is available in Europe as calcium serdolit.

Resins continue to exchange cations in the gut for up to one week after they have been taken orally, so that *hypokalaemia* may be a problem requiring treatment a few days after the problem of hyperkalaemia has been overcome.

Cation exchange resins can be given *per rectum as enemata* because of the high K concentration in the faecal fluid in the colon. The final K^+

exchange takes place in the colon. This has been dealt with in the paragraphs dealing with physiology of K and the intestinal tract. Sorbitol is sometimes given with K-exalate. Sorbitol by itself gets rid of K in the form of diarrhoea, 1 litre containing about 20 mEq of K and 90−100 mEq of Na. Sorbitol with Kay-exalate prevents the latter exchanging for K in the colon.

5.   To be on the safe side in renal failure patients, after the glucose and insulin has been given, and while awaiting the beginning of the action of cation-exchange resins it is wise **to commence dialysis with potassium free solution to remove** K from the body. The total amount of K in the ECF in only about 100 mEq if the plasma level is 7 mEq. Dialysis prevents the unpleasant surprise of finding hyperkalaemia to have recurred about 12 hours after treatment with glucose and insulin. Dietary therapy should be instituted in patients with hyperkalaemia and chronic renal failure by giving a diet with not more than 30 mEq of potassium in it. Usually 10−30 mEq of K will appear in the faeces each day in renal failure so that this small oral load may be within the excretory capability of the gut.

Question Where is most of the K^+ finally exchanged when a cation exchange resin is given?

Answer 1. In the stomach. Go on to **3.35**.
             2. In the small intestine. Go on to **3.33**.
             3. In the colon. Go on to **3.36**.

3.33   Your answer—K^+ exchange finally takes place in the small intestine.
      No. K^+ exchange finally takes place in the colon. You have not read **3.32** carefully. Read it again.

3.34   Your answer—potassium hydroxide.
      This is a ridiculous guess. Potassium hydroxide is a corrosive alkali and fatal to take. You are not good at guessing, so you should read **3.29** again.

3.35   Your answer—K^+ exchange finally takes place in the stomach.
      No you are guessing. Potassium is secreted into the stomach but this is not the final site of exchange unless you vomit the resin. You should read **3.32** again.

3.36   Your answer—In the colon.
      You are correct.

Physiology of potassium in the gastro-intestinal tract. The intestinal tract is very roughly comparably to nephron in that the small intestine is like the proximal tubule, where there is predominant absorption of potassium, and the large intestine like the distal nephron, where there is K secretion. Thus particularly on the left side of the colon and in the rectum there is predominant secretion of potassium. Small intestinal secretions contain $10-30$ mEq of potassium per litre, and similar amounts of potassium or larger may be found in the gastric secretions. Vomiting or prolonged diarrhoea, sometimes caused by laxative abuse, results in a loss of potassium from the body which may be serious and cause depletion of total body stores of potassium, and accompanying hypokalaemic alkalosis. In all cases of pyloric stenosis such total body K losses may amount to several hundred milliequivalents and require replenishment together with the more obvious sodium loss *before* operation. Similarly in severe diarrhoea such as caused by idiopathic stearrhoea, Crohn's disease, or ulcerative colitis, potassium loss may be very extensive and result in tetany, muscular weakness, ileus and ECG changes, the symptoms responding readily to replenishment.

The effect of potassium on the resin–angiotensin–aldosterone axis has of late received some attention. It is becoming clear that low levels of K intake which are sufficient to cause K depletion result in an increase in circulating renin activity, and angiotensin II levels. The converse, potassium loading, causes a rise in plasma aldosterone levels either without any change in plasma renin activity (PRA) or angiotensin II levels, or with some increase in PRA.

Papillomata of the lower colon and rectum may secrete large quantities of potassium and so cause hypokalaemia with depletion of whole body potassium stores. If a solution of saline is introduced as an enema into the colon and retained for an hour, on evacuation after an hour it will be found that much of the sodium has been reabsorbed and replaced by potassium, and that chloride has been reabsorbed and replaced by bicarbonate. If the operation of uretero-sigmoidostomy is performed (the ureters being transplanted to the sigmoid), then there is reabsorption of sodium and chloride from the urine in the colon, with secretion into it of potassium and bicarbonate. This results in a state of hypokalaemic acidosis, caused by the loss of potassium and bicarbonate, with high plasma chloride levels. The immediate preventive therapy is to prevent urine accumulating in the sigmoid colon and rectum by emptying the contents of the bowel as often as possible, and at a maximal interval of two hours, so that as little time as possible is left for ion exchange of the urine in the colon. Of course potassium citrate can be given orally in sufficient quantity to neutralize the acidosis and hypokalaemia. It would seem, however, that this operation is becoming progressively less frequent, and reimplantation of the ureters into an ileal conduit is preferable, where the urine can drain externally into a sealed receptacle and not be in prolonged contact with mucosa capable of absorption. However the same complication can occur with ileal conduit as with ureterosigmoidostomy. I see them frequently.

Now answer the question.

Question In a patient with ureterosigmoidostomy would you expect hypokalaemia or hyperkalaemia?

Answer 1. Hyperkalaemia. Go on to **3.37**.
       2. Hypokalaemia. Go on to **3.39**.

3.37 Your answer—hyperkalaemia.

You are guessing. If you had read **3.36** correctly you would not have made such a choice. Hyperkalaemia is not found in the run-of-the-mill case after ureterosigmoidostomy. Go back to **3.37**.

3.38 Your answer—no potassium.

No. You have not paid adequate attention to **3.36** and **3.39**. If you cannot concentrate try and get away from distractions and read both **3.36** and **3.39** again.

3.39 Your answer—hypokalaemia.

You are correct. In severe uraemia there is an increase in plasma aldosterone secretion, and this is important because it contributes to an increased potassium concentration in faecal water, and thus a maximal potassium excretion in the faeces in these patients, as shown by Wrong and his colleagues using a PVP (polyvinylpyrrolidine) filled dialysis membrane bag taken orally and analyzed after passage per rectum, where the Na/K is considerably lower in uraemia than in normal man. Remember that in man the small intestinal secretions contain 10—30 mEq of K per litre. It is known from anephric dialysis patients that potassium influences directly renal renin release and angiotensin II. However, if there is *very severe potassium depletion*, aldosterone secretion is *inhibited* and one gets high renin, low plasma K and low plasma aldosterone levels. This is associated with the loss of a urine rich in Na^+ and Cl^-, despite hypokalaemia.

Sweat potassium loss may be considerable, but is increased after administration of aldosterone and in the naturally acclimatized subject.

Diminished total body reserves of potassium are found in subjects working in hot desert conditions, but are by no means constant.

Now answer the question:

Question How much potassium is found in the small intestinal secretions?

Answer 1. No potassium at all. Go on to **3.38**.
          2. 10—30 mEq/l. Go on to **3.40**.
          3. 30—100 mEq/l. Go on to **3.41**.

3.40   Your answer— 10—30 mEq/l of potassium.

You are correct. Potassium levels in the plasma are also controlled by
aldosterone even in the absence of the kidneys, as shown in anephric
patients who are maintained alive by regular haemodialysis. Aldosterone
is secreted in response to potassium loading and is responsible for the
entry of potassium into the cells of these patients. Thus potassium levels
in the plasma are *partially controlled* by aldosterone secretion, with plasma
potassium influencing the release of aldosterone from the adrenal cortex.
Of course in the presence of normal kidneys high potassium levels also
stimulate the release of renin which results in the increased production of
Angiotensin II. The latter reaches the adrenal cortex and stimulates
increased secretion of aldosterone which results in increased sodium
reabsorption particularly in the distal tubule, and K secretion.

The effect of insulin and glucose on potassium uptake by the liver has
been shown to occur in isolated liver preparations in the *absence* of glucose
and is thus primarily an *insulin-mediated* mechanism of controlling plasma
potassium levels; indeed as in the case of aldosterone there may be positive
feedback loop, mediated by serum K levels, of insulin release. In Bartter's
syndrome there is severe hypokalaemic alkalosis *without hypertension*,
with highly elevated plasma renin levels and plasma aldosterone levels,
with an *inadequate* arteriolar response to angiotensin as the cause of the
lack of hypertension. In many patients with this syndrome there is a degree
of renal wasting i.e. inability to conserve sodium and this may be the cause
of contraction of ECF with a lower plasma volume and be a stimulus to
renin secretion. Histologically there is enlargement of the juxta-glomerular
apparatus. Remember that in Bartter's syndrome the prostaglandin
synthetase inhibitor indomethacin causes reversal of most of the biochemical abnormalities, so that the disease is presumably related to
abnormal renal prostaglandin metabolism at some stage in its pathogenesis. In some patients a condition of low plasma renin with low plasma

aldosterone and hyperkalaemia is present. (This is known as Type IV RTA —see Chapter 7.) It appears that the hyperkalaemia is a result of the reduced aldosterone secretion and absence of the aldosterone feedback loop described above which controls plasma K levels. It is particularly common in diabetic patients.

Now answer the question:

Question A patient is found to have a serum potassium level of 7.2 mEq/litre with a serum creatinine level of 1.0 mg/100 ml and a serum sodium of 137 mEq/l. Plasma aldosterone levels are low, and plasma renin levels are subnormal. What is the diagnosis?

Answer 1. Bartter's syndrome. Go on to **3.43**.
           2. Hyporeninic hypoaldosteronism or Type IV RTA. Go on to **3.45**.

3.41 Your answer—30 to 100 mEq/ l.
     You are guessing. This figure was not in **3.36** or **3.39**. Go back and read both **3.36** and **3.39** carefully.

3.42   Your answer—statement 1 is true, 2 and 3 are false.
     So you think potassium is the main cation of the ECF. How wrong can you get? Use a little intelligence. You seem to have forgotten the contents of both this chapter and that a Chapter 2 on sodium. Start at the beginning of Chapter 3 again.

3.43 Your answer—Bartter's syndrome.
     Your answer is incorrect. It is purely the result of guessing and not concentrating when you were reading **3.40**. In any case the point about Bartter's syndrome was made earlier on. Go back and read **3.40** again.

3.44   Your answer—statement 2 is true, 1 and 3 are false.
     You are correct. You can go on to Chapter 4. If you want to look up pertinent monographs on potassium the following monographs are recommended:

Brenner B. and Stern J. (Eds) (1978) *Acid Base and Potassium Homeo-stasis.* Churchill Livingstone, London.
Wright F. S. (1977) Sites and mechanisms of potassium transport along the renal tubule. *Kidney International.* **11**, 415−432.
Silva P., Hayslett J. P. and Epstein F. H. (1973) Chronic K^+ adaptations.

Table 3.44.   Emergency treatment of hyperkalaemia

IV   10 ml of 10 per cent $CaCl_2$ in 5 minutes
IV   100 mEq of $NaHCO_3$ in 5 minutes
IV   insulin 20 units and 50 ml of 50 per cent dextrose in 5 minutes
Rectally   30 g of Kay-exalate
Orally   20 g to 8 hourly of Kay-exalate
Then—Dialyse against zero K dialysate as soon as this can be done, and within 4 hours

Role of Na, K APTase. *J. Clin. Invest.* **52**, 2665–2671.

Maxwell and Kleemans monograph on *Clinical Disorders of Fluid and Electrolyte Metabolism.*

Schreir R. *Renal and Electrolyte Disorders* (Little Brown, Boston) is highly recommended.

This is still the most readable and scholarly source. Before you leave this chapter look at Table 3.44. Make sure you know it.

3.45   Your answer—hyporeninic hypoaldosteronism or Type IV RTA.

You are correct. Now look at the following statements and choose the correct answer:

Statement 1.   Potassium is the main cation of ECF.

Statement 2.   No symptoms of K deficiency appear until there is a deficit of 10–30 per cent of body potassium.

Statement 3.   Oral KCl tablets do not cause intestinal ulceration.

Choose the correct answer from the following:

Answer   1.   Statement 1 is true, 2 and 3 are false. Go on to **3.42**.
         2.   Statement 2 is true, 1 and 3 are false. Go on to **3.44**.
         3.   Statement 3 is true, 1 and 2 are false. Go on to **3.46**.
         4.   All the statements are true. Go on to **3.47**.

3.46   Your answer—statement 3 is true, 1 and 2 are false.

Well you can't have been concentrating very well in this chapter. Start again at **3.1**.

3.47   Your answer—all statements are true.

You are guessing, there is no point in fooling yourself. Start again at **3.1** and work through.

Time for this chapter: $1\frac{1}{2}$ hours

Chapter 4
Calcium

4.1   Calcium is a cation of great importance: it is the major cation in the skeleton, responsible for many of the unusual and specific properties of bone, and at the same time is an important constituent of the intracellular and extracellular fluids. It is of major importance in nerve conduction and neuromuscular conduction potentials, and in normal health its concentration in the ECF is rigidly controlled by a very complicated hormonal control mechanism. This fascinating cation has been the subject of remarkable discoveries of late as the details of the hormonal role of vitamin D are discovered.

1100 g of calcium is found in the human adult body. This figure comes both from direct chemical measurement in the cadaver, which has been performed in a small number of subjects, and from neutron activation studies. The chemical method has been described in the chapters on sodium and potassium and I assume that you can recall this simple, method of dissolving the body in acid and measuring the calcium content of the solution. Let us look at other methods for measuring total body calcium in the *live* human being; the most frequently used of these is known as the 'Neutron Activation' technique. In this technique a beam of neutrons from a neutron source, such as Plutonium and Americium or from a Neutron generator is directed uniformly over the body of the subject, in a harmless dose (equivalent to less than a chest X ray's irradiation). The neutrons penetrate the tissues and are chosen to have sufficient energy to react with calcium nuclei and make them radioactive, emitting γ rays. These are then measured in a whole body counter, which has already been described in the previous chapter. It consists of a series of γ ray detectors usually large crystals of sodium iodide activated by thallium which are sensitive to gamma rays, converting them to photons which are then magnified by photomultiplier tubes. The crystals are set all round the body in the more expensive type of whole body counter; in a less costly model the subject is mechanically moved on a trolley through an array of crystals. The photomultiplier tubes are connected to multichannel analysers, and the radioactive calcium isotopes produced by the neutrons from stable calcium are counted with a moderately high degree of accuracy. Using a 'phantom' model of a body the machine can be calibrated and standardized to give answers in mmols of calcium in the body. Regularly, however, the machine can be used to give answers in non-absolute units and the results compared over a period of months with repeat measurements to give percentage changes in total body calcium content. The whole body counter/neutron activation method is probably accurate to 5 per cent in most hands, although the most advanced designs are thought to be accurate to ± 2.5 per cent. Their main use is in detecting *changes* in whole body calcium and not in absolute measurements.

Question How accurate is neutron activation estimation of calcium?

Answer 1. To within ± 0.1 per cent. Go on to **4.3**.
          2. To within 2.5 to 5.0 per cent. Go on to **4.5**.
          3. 10.0 per cent. Go on to **4.7**.

4.2   What are you reading this for? Follow instructions or do not waste your time reading this book.

4.3   Your answer—accurate to within 0.1 per cent.
No. You are guessing. This is no way to learn. Go back to **4.1** and start again. However, if you are distracted and cannot prevent it, stop fooling yourself and aimlessly looking at the page.

4.4   Your answer—10 per cent.
No. 1089 g out of the body's total of 1100 g is found in the skeleton. You are not concentrating. Read **4.5** again.

4.5   Your answer—2.5 to 5.0 per cent.
You are correct. It depends on where you work. Dr. S. Cohn's laboratory at Brookhaven, New York, is possibly the most accurate at 2.5 per cent, but most have a 5.0 per cent error.
Exchangeable calcium (Ca_E) by use of oral ^{47}Ca cannot be meaningfully and adequately measured because of the increasing value obtained if the time interval for equilibration is increased from 1, to 2, 3, 4, 5, 6, or 7 days. Daily collection of 24 hour urine collections for all this time would require admission to a hospital and often is frought with 'accidents' where a sample is lost and so a day's collection is incomplete and the entire experiment has to be scrapped. The increasing Ca_E value is due to the increasing penetration, with time, of deeper layers of the bone crystal. In practice no one bothers to measure Ca_E. An alternative method of

measuring calcium in the body is by measuring the calcium present in chosen individual bones, usually limb and vertebral bones. There are 2 methods in widespread use: the first method is by taking X ray films, under rigidly standardized conditions, of the arms and hands using a standard aluminium stepped wedge (which has been calibrated against bone mineral). The density of the bone on the X ray film is measured with a densitometer and changes of less than 5–10 per cent can be measured accurately. Similarly bone density in the distal parts of the limbs can be measured by the absorption of gamma rays by the bone. A gamma ray source, usually radio-iodine, is positioned under the limb and the collimated crystal detector measures what rays come through the bone. In both these methods the major bone density to X rays and γ rays is due to the calcium salts in the bone i.e. to the bone's mineral content, predominantly calcium.

The total amount of calcium in the body is about 1100 g in the adult. Of this 1089 g or 99 per cent is found in the skeleton, 10 g is found to be in the non-skeletal intracellular compartment, and 1 g is found in the extracellular space. Look at these figures again: Remember 1 per cent of calcium is *extra*skeletal.

Question What percentage of total body calcium is found in the skeleton? Don't look back at what you've read. Choose the correct answer.

Answer 1. 10 per cent. Go on to **4.4**.
2. 99 per cent. Go on to **4.8**.
3. 1 per cent. Go on to **4.9**.

4.6 Your answer—protein-bound calcium.
No. you can hardly be reading carefully. Protein-bound calcium is *not* active in nerve conduction. It is ionized calcium that is important. You should have remembered that this from your physiology studies, even if you did not read **4.8**.

4.7 Your answer—10.0 per cent.
No. You are guessing. You have just started the chapter—there is no real reason for not learning properly unless you are being distracted. If you cannot give reading your full attention, stop now. Start **4.1** again when you can read in an undistracted manner.

4.8 Your answer—99 per cent of body calcium is in the skeleton.
You are correct. Let us look at the extracellular space first. In the plasma, calcium is found in a total concentration of 9–11 mg/100 ml

($2.25-2.75 \, mmol \, l^{-1}$) 40 per cent is protein bound, in the main to serum albumin. The carriage of calcium on albumin is of particular importance because it is necessary to correct calcium concentrations in plasma for changes in serum albumin level to determine whether the calcium level is normal. Look at the nomogram which gives an idea of the size of the correction necessary. Remember this is only a rough correction.

If you are away from a nomogram then a rough guide is a depression of $0.2 \, mmol \, l^{-1}$ (0.8 mg/100 ml) for every g/100 ml fall in albumin concentration. Of the non-albumin bound calcium about $1.25 \, mmol \, l^{-1}$ (5 mg/100 ml) is in the form of ionized calcium, and $0.125 \, mmol \, l^{-1}$ (0.5 mg) is in the form of diffusable, but non-ionized, calcium principally in the form of citrate and phosphate. The plasma level of ionized calcium is of major physiological importance as the integrity of neuromuscular transmission is dependent on plasma *ionized calcium* levels. The extracellular fluid outside the vascular tree contains very little protein so that the protein bound 40 per cent of plasma calcium is not present, and the total calcium found in the tissue fluid is in the order of $1.25-1.3 \, mmol \, l^{-1}$ (5 to 6 mg per

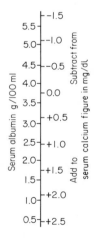

Albumin binding correction

Nomogram for correction of serum
calcium by serum albumin figure
(modified from Dr A.Miller,
Courtauld Institute,
Middlesex Hospital,
London)

Fig. 4.8   Calcium serum albumin nomogram.

100 ml) *1.1—1.25 mmol* (4.5 to 5 mg) of which are ionized, the remainder being divided between diffusable non-ionized calcium and protein bound calcium.

Ionized calcium falls as the plasma pH rises and vice versa. If we look at intracellular calcium it is much lower in concentration that extracellular calcium. Intracellular calcium should be thought of *not* as a homogeneous entity, but as differing in concentration and physical and chemical forms in the various subcellular compartments. Although calcium concentration in 'ICF' is lower than plasma it is particularly low in the cytosol and its concentration is controlled by release of calcium from the mitochondria. The calcium concentrations in the cytosol measured by fluorescent materials or metalloprotein indicators are ionic calcium measurements. One thing is certain—that in health ionic calcium and total calcium levels are both lower in the cytosol than in ECF.

Question What is the calcium fraction responsible for integrity of neuromuscular transmission?

Answer 1. Protein bound calcium. Go on to **4.6**.
        2. Ionized calcium. Go on to **4.10**.
        3. Diffusible calcium. Go on to **4.12**.

4.9 Your answer—1 per cent.

No. 1 per cent of calcium is extraskeletal. Therefore you have not concentrated while reading **4.5**. Read it again.

4.10 Your answer—ionized calcium.

You are correct. The diet contains about *20 to 25 mmol* (800 g—1000 mg) per day of calcium, but this is mainly dependent on the amount of milk and cheese eaten. Of the calcium found in the faeces some *5 mmol* (200 mg) can be shown by tracer studies to have been *secreted from* the blood *into* the GI tract. *5—7.5 mmol* (200—300 mg) of this mixture of the food and the calcium secreted calcium is absorbed and the remaining calcium is excreted in the faeces.

Intestinal absorption of calcium is fairly complicated. It is dependent on the presence of a specific calcium-binding protein in the cells of the small intestine. This protein seems to be produced in response to a stimulus produced by the presence of 1:25 $(OH)_2$ Vitamin D_3, and 24:25 $(OH)_2$ Vit. D_3. These hormones are thought to cause an increase in RNA responsible for the ultimate synthesis of the calcium carrier proteins. Intestinal absorption of calcium is also dependent on the presence of parathyroid hormone which induces the formation of 1:25 $(OH)_2 D_3$ from 25 OH D_3 as well as the presence of corticosteroids such as hydro-cortisone. The method of interaction between these several hormonal factors including calcitonin remains to be clarified completely.

Phytic acid is found in diets in many parts of the world where unleavened bread is eaten. Phytic acid is present in cereals such as wheat. Yeast forms phytase, an enzyme which destroys phytic acid (inositol hexaphosphate). Unleavened bread is not made with yeast so phytic acid remains in the bread. Phytic acid is capable of chelating calcium, mag-nesium, zinc and iron. Thus in India, Iran and the Near East unleavened bread can chelate much of the dietary calcium (which is low anyway) and lead to osteomalacia and possibly also to osteoporosis. Large quantities of magnesium present in the gut may interfere with calcium absorption.

Question How much calcium is secreted into the intestine from the blood?

Answer   1. *25 mmol* (1000 mg). Go on to **4.13**.
2. *5 mmol* (200 mg). Go on to **4.15**.
3. *37.5 mmol* (1500 mg). Go on to **4.16**.

4.11   Your answer—absorption of calcium is increased.

You are correct. Hypercalcaemia is defined as elevation of the plasma calcium level. The normal level is *2.25 to 2.75 mmol l^{-1}* (9 to 11.0 mg/100 ml) Results of plasma calcium over 10.5 mg/100 ml should be regarded as suspicious and repeated. It is a good plan to repeat abnormal tests to confirm their abnormality unless there are alternatives methods for cor-roborating the abnormal result. One of the most important reasons for this is that nowadays with automated apparatus not infrequently one sample gets out of step and misidentified and the clinician is supplied with the results from an incorrectly identified patient. It is the equivalent in medi-cine of the surgeon's amputating a leg in a patient who has been anaes-thetized because of appendicitis—and no less serious. So first repeat the test quickly and also check all results of plasma calcium over *2.6 mmol l^{-1}* (10.5 mg/100 ml). Do not forget that an elevated plasma calcium level may result from excessive stasis in the taking of blood sample. It is best to repeat the test without a tourniquet. Also use serum, not heparinized plasma, because the heparin has been implicated in false reduction of the calcium concentration due to the formation of calcium—heparin complexes which precipitate. Now let us assume that the high plasma calcium result is confirmed. Hypercalcaemia comes about as a result of either increased bone catabolism, abnormally high calcium absorption or decreased ability

Table 4.11. Causes of hypercalcaemia (after Popovtzer)

Hyperparathyroidism, Primary
Secondary
   Malabsorption and vitamin D deficiency
   Chronic renal failure
   Following kidney transplantation (Tertiary)
Neoplastic Diseases
   Malignant tumour with metastases to the bones
   Tumours secreting parathyroid hormone-like substances
   Tumours secreting humoral nonparathyroid-like substances (i.e. prostaglandins)
   Multiple myeloma and other lymphoproliferative diseases—'osteoclast-activating factor'
Vitamin D intoxication
Vitamin A intoxication
Hyperthyroidism
Adrenocortical insufficiency
Immobilization in Pager's disease
Milk—Alkali syndrome
Hypercalcaemia associated with acute renal failure
Thiazide-induced hypercalcaemia
Use of calcium-ion exchange resins
Hypophosphatasia
Infantile hypercalcaemia

Learn this list. Write it out 5 times with the book closed. Don't go on until you know it.

to excrete calcium. Let us look at each in turn. Look at Table 4.11. Learn it. Now let us look at the factors. First of all the plasma calcium level is elevated in hyperparathyroidism, and it has been suggested that repeated measurement of the plasma calcium to detect occasional elevation of plasma calcium is the best test to detect cases of hyperparathyroidism in the renal stone clinic population. Hypercalcaemia is frequent in primary hyperparathyroidism often accompanied by hyperchloridaemia due to the renal tubular acidosis caused by parathyroid hormone as Muldowney has shown. Serum calcium levels as high as *4.25 mmol l^{-1}* (17 mg/100 ml) occur in primary hyperparathyrodism and become higher with immobilization if there is a pathological fracture complicating a brown bone cyst.

Hypercalcaemia can be caused by any factor causing bone destruction: These include hyperparathyroidism (usually primary, but sometimes secondary), excessive vitamin D therapy, or therapy with one of its metabolites such as $1,25(OH)_2$ D3, $1\ \alpha OHD_3$, or $25\ (OH)D_3$, or AT 10 (dihydrotachysterol). Vitamin D intoxication, hyperthyroidism, metastatic bone disease, particularly bronchial carcinoma producing parathyroid like hormone, prostatic carcinoma, sarcoid, myeloma, immobilization in Paget's disease, administration of thiazide diuretics, spurious elevation due to stasis before taking various blood samples and contamination of blood due to use of cork stoppers. In addition milk—alkali syndrome, and recovery from acute renal failure particularly due to acute rhabdomyolysis are associated with hypercalcaemia. In hypothyroidism injection of quite small calcium loads may cause hypercalcaemia. In adrenal insufficiency hypercalcaemia may develop which responds well to steroids. In infants, idiopathic hypercalcaemia was at one time common due to excessive amounts of vitamin D being given to infants in the prevention of rickets. In hypophosphatasia, an inherited rare disease, hypercalcaemia may be found. Calcium containing ion-exchange resins may cause hypercalcaemia if given to patients with good renal function or to whose who are on haemodialysis. Hypercalcaemia after transplantation is often due to tertiary hyperparathyroidism i.e. an adenoma which is unmasked after transplantation. It may disappear spontaneously 6 months post transplantation.

Hypercalcaemia can be treated by intravenous sodium phosphate infusion, with a resultant fall in plasma calcium levels but detailed therapy will be discussed later. The cause of this fall in plasma calcium levels after phosphate infusion is probably too rapid to be due to a decrease in PTH secretion causing a fall in liberation of calcium from the bones; it cannot be due to a renal effect because it is present in renal failure. It has been suggested that it is a result of a calcium phosphate colloid being formed and sequestered in the liver and released slowly later. Certainly one of the dangers of this form of therapy is metastatic calcification due to calcium phosphate deposition in the arterial walls. A frequent question asked by students is 'what is the cause of the frequently seen reciprocal relationship between plasma levels of calcium and phosphorus'? It is possibly due to a complex interrelationship between the hormones responsible for calcium and phosphorus homeostasis, i.e. parathyroid hormone, calcitonin and $1:25$ and $24:25$ $(OH)_2$ Vitamin D, and the entire story is probably not yet known.

Thus there are many patients in whom the reciprocal relationship does not exist i.e. patients with high plasma calcium and high plasma phosphorus levels in renal failure with predominant hyperparathyroidism. They develop metastatic calcification when the plasma calcium $\times$ phosphorus product (expressed in mg/100 ml and *not* in SI units) rise above 70.

Question What is the plasma chloride level in primary hyperparathyroidism?

Answer 1. Increased. Go on to **4.18**.
2. Normal. Go on to **4.20**.
3. Decreased. Go on to **4.22**.

4.12 Your answer—diffusible calcium.
You are partly correct in that ionized calcium is the greater part of diffusable calcium. However you would have picked the correct answer— ionized calcium—if you were concentrating. Go back to **4.8** and read it carefully.

4.13 Your answer—*25 mmol* (1000 mg) of calcium is secreted into the intestine.
No. This is the total amount of calcium in the average diet. You have guessed badly. Read **4.13** again and concentrate this time.

4.14 Your answer—the amount of calcium reabsorbed decreased. You are guessing. Read **4.15**.

4.15 You answer—*5 mmol* (200 mg) calcium.
You are correct. Renal failure is associated with an impaired calcium absorption due to impairment of renal synthesis of 1:25 $(OH)_2$ Vit.D_3 and 24:25 $(OH)_2$ Vit.D_3 which are responsible for the synthesis of calcium carrier proteins in the small intestine. This impairment of synthesis is due to lack of the l-hydroxylase or 24 hydroxylase enzymes which are present in normal kidneys. In acute renal failure in man and dog there is an increase in brain cortical calcium, as Massry and Arieff have shown. Possibly the uraemic cerebral metabolic changes with low frequency EEF waves are due to the calcium deposited in the cerebral cortex due to massively elevated parathyroid hormone levels in acute renal failure.
Urinary excretion of calcium on a normal diet is less than 300 mg/day (*7.5 mmol*) in man and less than 250 mg/day (*6 mmol*) in women *in health*. Renal handling of calcium is such that only the diffusible and ionized calcium can be filtered, the albumin bound calcium being of necessity unable to traverse the glomerular filter. Thus of every 100 ml of GFR plasma filtered per minute only about *1.4 mmol* l^{-1} (5.5 mg per cent) of calcium are filtered and *1–1.25 mmol* l^{-1} (4–5 per cent) remains protein-

bound and unfiltered. In the proximal tubule 50—70 per cent of the filtered calcium is reabsorbed. This proximal calcium reabsorption is linked in a somewhat loose way to the absorption of sodium and magnesium. Expansion of ECF by mineralocorticoid administration causes increased proximal tubular rejection of sodium, magnesium and calcium. On the other hand after a few days therapy with thiazide diuretics calcium excretion falls although there may be a rise in plasma calcium levels. This fact is used in the treatment of idiopathic hypocalcuria when small doses of hydrochlorothiazide may radically reduce excretion of calcium and significantly reduce urinary stone formation. 10 per cent of filtered calcium is reabsorbed in the distal tubule and the remaining 20—40 per cent in the thick ascending part of the loop of Henle.

Parathyroid hormone causes an increase in the filtered load of calcium by its hypercalcaemic action, and pari passu with this an increased *tubular reabsorption* of calcium. The increase in filtered load is so great that despite the increased tubular reabsorption is unable to absorb the increased filtered load and there is such an increase in the amount of non-reabsorbed calcium, that the result is an increased calcium-excretion in the urine. The hypercalcaemia is a result of both an increase in bone resorption (see Fig. 4.15) and an increase in absorption of calcium. The

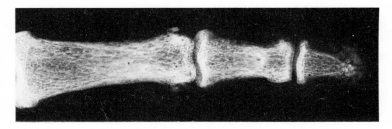

Fig. 4.15a

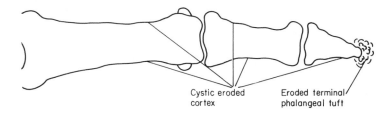

Cystic eroded   Eroded terminal
cortex   phalangeal tuft

Fig. 4.15b

tubular reabsorption of ionized calcium is more efficient than that of complexed calcium, so that urinary calcium is 20 per cent ionized and 80 per cent complexed. Urinary calcium is mainly bound by citrate 60 per cent at pH 7 and only 40 per cent at pH 5. Acidosis is associated with an increase in urinary calcium excretion, as is ethanol or glucose administration. Administration intravenously of phosphate salts causes a fall in urinary calcium due to an increase in tubular reabsorption. This is probably not mediated by the parathyroid gland, because the same response occurs in parathyroidectomized vitamin D treated dogs. Phosphate depletion causes hypercalciuria, again by a mechanism of reduced tubular reabsorption of calcium.

Question What is the effect of PTH on tubular reabsorption of calcium.

Answer 1. Increased. Go on to **4.11**.
2. Decreased. Go on to **4.14**.
3. No effect. Go on to **4.17**.

4.16 Your answer—*37.5 mmol* (1500 mg) of calcium secreted into the intestine.
   You are not correct. This is a figure greater than the daily calcium intake. Read **4.13** again and do not guess, please.

4.17 Your answer—no effect.
   This is wrong. You are not concentrating again. Read **4.15** again but make sure you are not distracted.

4.18 Your answer—chloride is increased.
   You are correct. In secondary hyperparathyroidism due to renal disease the serum calcium is either normal or very mildly elevated until renal transplantation occurs, when the hypercalcaemia of so called 'tertiary hyperparathyroidism' is revealed, where there is frequently an autonomous parathyroid adenoma resulting from long-lasting parathyroid hypertrophy during the period of chronic haemodialysis. Primary hyperparathyroidism is usually associated with a high calcium, low plasma inorganic phosphorus level and raised plasma alkaline phosphatase and often an acidosis caused by the renal tubular effects of parathyroid hormone. There is an elevated PTH and usually a depressed tubular reabsorption of (TRP) phosphate.

TRP is defined as $\dfrac{\text{P filtered—P excreted in urine/min}}{\text{P filtered/min}}$.

The normal TRP is 0.85−0.90- and in primary hyperparathyroidism it is usually 0.60 or lower. Here are some typical results in primary hyperparathyroidism:

		Normal Value
Plasma calcium	15 mg/100 ml	9−11
	(3.75 mmol l⁻¹)	*(2.25−2.75 mmol l⁻¹)*
Plasma inorganic	1.5 mg/100 ml	3−4.5
phosphorus	*(0.5 mmol l⁻¹)*	*(1−1.5 mmol l⁻¹)*
Plasma alkaline		
phosphatase	20 KA units	5−12
TRP	0.60	0.85−0.90
Plasma chloride	*115 mmol l⁻¹*	95−105 mm/*l*
Blood urea	50 mg/100 ml	15−45 mg%
	(8.3 mmol l⁻¹)	*(2.5−7.5 mmol l⁻¹)*

Hyperparathyroidism secondary to renal disease can be differentiated from primary hyperparathyroidism by:

1. the history of primary renal disease in secondary hyperparathyroidism;
2. decreased renal function as shown by a low creatinine clearance;
3. by normal or slightly elevated plasma calcium levels in the presence of variable plasma inorganic P levels which may be low, normal or raised.

In the earlier stages of renal failure there is a normal plasma inorganic P level or occasionally a minimally lowered one, but as renal failure advances plasma inorganic P levels rise. Parathyroid hormone levels are elevated. TRP is diminished as in primary hyperparathyroidism. Brown tumours are rarer in the bones in secondary hyperparathyroidism, but do occur. Thus it is clear that the easiest way of diagnosing secondary hyperparathyroidism is by means of the history. Indeed as the late Lord Platt pointed out in another context—more than 90 per cent of correct diagnoses can be made by letting the patient talk, a small percentage on physical examination, and an even smaller percentage on biochemical and other tests. This is true of most of the patients you will see in your clinical career as a doctor, but not true of many electrolyte problems which are only unravellable by means of sophisticated laboratory tests. A set of results of some common biochemical tests in renal hyperparathyroidism is shown below.

		SI units	mg/100 ml
Plasma calcium (*2.5 mmol l⁻¹*)	11.0 mg/100 ml		
Plasma inorganic (*2.3 mmol l⁻¹*)	7.0 mg/100 ml		
Plasma alkaline phosphatase	25 KA units		
Blood urea (*33 mmol l⁻¹*)	200 mg/100 ml		
TRP	0.50		

Write in the normal
values below

Now write in the normal values in the column on the right.

Good. Of late a further requirement has been added to the diagnosis of hyperparathyroidism. This is the TmP/GFR and will be discussed in detail in the chapter on phosphorus metabolism.

Question A patient has the following results:
bone X ray changes of hyperparathyroidism. Plasma biochemistry as follows:

Serum calcium 7.5 mg/100 ml (*1.9 mmol l⁻¹*).
Serum inorganic P. 8.0 mg/100 ml (*2.7 mmol l⁻¹*).
Serum creatinine 11 mg/100 ml (*1 mmol l⁻¹*).
Serum chloride 101 mEq/l. (*101 mmol l⁻¹*).

What is the patient suffering from?

Answer 1. Primary hyperparathyroidism. Go on to **4.19**.
           2. Secondary hyperparathyroidism. Go on to **4.21**.

4.19 Your answer—primary hyperparathyroidism.
    No you have not got the message in **4.18**. Read it again then answer the question.

4.20 Your answer—The plasma chloride level is normal.
    You are wrong. There is an acidosis due to high levels of PTH. Hence plasma bicarbonate levels are depressed and the anion gap not being increased, plasma chloride is increased. Read **4.11** again. It contains many parts that you may have missed.

4.21   Your answer—secondary hyperparathyroidism.

You are correct. Hypercalcaemia is commonly found in malignant disease. It may be the result of actual destruction of the skeleton by widespread bony metastases, or due to production by the tumour of parathyroid-hormone *like* substances which react immunologically with the antibodies to parathyroid hormone and so can be detected on PTH radioimmunoassay of the serum. Metastases which riddle the skeleton and cause hypercalcaemia by bone destruction include carcinoma of breast, thyroid, prostrate, kidney and bronchus and multiple myeloma is particularly associated with hypercalcaemia and bony erosion. Some leukaemias infiltrate the skeleton and so do lymphomas, all capable of causing hypercalcaemia by bone destruction with liberation of calcium from the bone in excess of calcium homeostatic mechanisms to deal with it, so that plasma calcium is elevated. Apparently in some malignancies the bone destruction is mediated by prostaglandins which are liberated locally by tumour cells and erode the bone. In carcinoma of the bronchus, in particular, where there are no bony metastases, there is likely to be a PTH-like hormone in circulation produced by the tumour. Common tumours other than bronchus producing PTH-like material are tumours of kidney, ovary and colon. In tumour metastases causing skeletal breakdown due to tumour cells eroding bone, the biochemical profile is likely to be:

> Plasma calcium *3.1 mmol l^{-1}*   (12.5 mg/100 ml)
> Plasma inorganic
> phosphorus *1.2 mmol l^{-1}*   (3.5 mg/100 ml)
> Plasma alkaline
> phosphatase   25 KA units.

In patients with tumours secreting a PTH like substance the biochemical profile is like that in primary hyperparathyroidism with the real diagnosis being made by history, physical examination and appropriate X ray studies to demonstrate the primary tumour and subsequent biopsy to give an unequivocal histological diagnosis. In myeloma there is an osteoclast stimulating substance.

Question A 45 year old patient is admitted to hospital with anorexia, dysphagia and constipation. Physical examination shows a chronically ill man, with an increased thirst and polyuria. Urine has an osmolality of 170 mOsm/kg. Faecal fat normal. Serum albumin 4.5 g/100 ml. Serum calcium *3.5 mmol l^{-1}* or 14 mg/100 ml. Serum creatinine 0.5 mg/100 ml. Serum inorganic phosphate *1.3 mmol l^{-1}* or 4 mg/100 ml. Serum PTH normal. Serum chloride 101 mEq *mmol l^{-1}*. IVP shows a space occupying lesion in the upper 2/3 of the right kidney. TRP = 85 per cent. What diagnosis would you make?

1. Primary hyperparathyroidism. Go on to **4.28**.
2. Secondary hyperparathyroidism. Go on to **4.26**.
3. Bone metastases with hypercalcaemia. Go on to **4.24**.

4.22   Your answer—decreased plasma chloride levels are found.

You are wrong. In primary hyperparathyroidism the high PTH levels cause an increased renal tubular loss of bicarbonate, so that a normal anion gap acidosis occurs, with increased plasma chloride levels. So it appears you have been guessing. That is pointless. Try and remove distractions or stop learning until you can concentrate. Go back and read **4.11** again.

4.23   You should not be reading this. Follow the instructions.

4.24   Your answer—bone metastases with hypercalcaemia.

You are correct. Good. The hypercalcaemia of vitamin D intoxication is the major toxic manifestation of vitamin D therapy. Because vitamin D_2 and D_3 are fat soluble and are stored in the liver where a 25 hydroxylase forms 25 hydroxyvitamin D_2 and 25 hydroxyvitamin D_3, it is apparent that vitamin D-induced hypercalcaemia will persist for *weeks*. On the other hand, the use of the newer synthetic derivatives of vitamin D such as 1 α hydroxycholecalciferol and 1,25 $(OH)_2$ vitamin D_3 causes hypercalcaemia persisting for only a *few days only*. Whenever one gives vitamin D or any of its derivatives repeated plasma calcium determinations should be performed to detect the first signs of hypercalcaemia. It should be remembered that in severe chronic renal failure with marked hypocalcaemia (say *1.25 mmol l^{-1}* or 5 mg/100 ml) and a high plasma phosphate level, (say *4 mmol l^{-1}* or 12 mg/100 ml) a rise of plasma calcium to *1.75 mmol l^{-1}* or 7 mg/100 ml will cause metastatic calcification (plasma Ca × P product = 84) so that *before* using vitamin D, or its products in hypocalcaemia, high plasma inorganic P levels should be reduced by oral administration of phosphate binders (such as calcium carbonate or aluminum hydroxide) or dialysis. Hypercalcaemia of vitamin D administration can be due to 2 mechanisms (1) bone resorption with liberation of calcium from the bone into the blood stream and (2) increased intestinal absorption of calcium. It is known that 1:25 dihydroxycholecalciferol causes an increase of mRNA in the intestinal mucosa, this mRNA being responsible for the production of calcium-binding protein which is necessary for the specific absorption of calcium from the intestinal contents. There is some evidence that two proteins binding calcium are made inside the intestinal cell. In sarcoidosis there is an apparent hypersensitivity to the intestinal calcium absorptive action of vitamin D, resulting in hypercalcaemia in *one third of patients with sarcoidosis*. The hypercalcaemia is highest when the 25 (OH) vitamin D_3 levels are highest, i.e. in the summer due to synthesis of 25 (OH) vitamin D_3 as a result of U.V. radiation of ergosterol in the skin forming cholecalciferol which is hydroxylated in the liver at the 25 position. Administration of corticosteroids in vitamin D intoxication and in sarcoidosis lowers the elevated plasma calcium. In hyperparathyroidism corticosteroids cause either no effect or the calcium lowering effect is not as dramatic as in sarcoidosis and vitamin D intoxication. Corticosteroids possible have this effect by blocking bone resorption, and thus can act as anti-vitamin D and anti-PTH agents. They may also help in severe hypercalcaemia associated with metastatic malignancies, but this is far less frequent than in vitamin D intoxication. In milk—alkali syndrome hypercalcaemia develops with nephrocalcinosis, renal failure, metastatic calcification and alkalosis, due to ingestion of large amounts of calcium in the antacids or in the milk which is taken as part of the therapeutic regimen. There is a good response of the hypercalcaemia to withdrawal of calcium from the diet, but some patients need corticosteroid therapy. Calcium-cycle ion exchange resins only rarely cause hypercalcaemia, but any patient on calcium resins or taking large quantities of calcium by mouth, should have his plasma calcium levels checked at weekly or two weekly intervals to determine whether hypercalcaemia is present, and if so to cut down the dose of calcium being given. Hyperthyroidism is an occasional cause of hypercalcaemia and must be excluded in all hypercalcaemias of unknown aetiology. Its frequency varies in different series, but it is probably less than 1 in 20 cases. The cause of hypercalcaemia is the greater degree of bone destruction in hyperthyroidism, liberating calcium and causing osteoporosis. Hypercalcuria is frequent, and far more frequent than hypercalcaemia: it is due to the excretion of the calcium liberated when bone is catabolized. Hypercalcuria leads to renal stone formation. In the differential diagnosis from hyperparathyroidism the tendency of hyperthyroidism to be associated with a normal or elevated serum inorganic P level is noteworthy. Administration of corticosteroids such as prednisone lowers the high plasma calcium levels in hyperthyroidism. In hypothyroidism, administration of calcium salts may cause marked hypercalcaemia due to the lack of utilization of calcium in bone formation. Bone formation is diminished in hypothyroidism.

Question A man with a peptic ulcer takes 8 teaspoonfuls of baking powder a day and 2 quarts of milk to obtain relief from his ulcer. His biochemical findings are as follows:

Serum calcium   14 mg/100 ml or *3.5 mmol l⁻¹*.
Serum inorganic phosphorus   7 mg/100 ml or *2.3 mmol l⁻¹*.
Blood urea nitrogen   53 mg/100 ml or *8.8 mmol l⁻¹*.
Alkaline phosphatase   25 KA units
Serum bicarbonate   33 mmol/l.

What is your diagnosis?

Answer 1. Primary hyperparathyroidism. Go on to **4.25**.
       2. Milk—alkali syndrome. Go on to **4.27**.
       3. Secondary hyperparathyroidism. Go on to **4.29**.

4.25 Your answer—primary hyperparathyroidism.
    No. First of all the biochemical picture is different. There is an acidosis in primary hyperparathyroidism and the phosphate is usually low although it may be normal in renal failure. In any case you are a poor guesser if you thought that the peptic ulcer therapy was put in as a non-sequitor. Go on and read **4.24** again.

4.26 Your answer—secondary hyperparathyroidism.
    How on earth do you come to that diagnosis? The patient has no evidence so you have guessed wrongly. Moreover you have not concentrated in reading **4.21**. Please read it again and try to shut the rest of the world, with its distractions, out of your mind. Think only of the words you are reading.

4.27 Your answer—milk—alkali syndrome.
    You are correct. Now answer the next question.

Question A 25 year old male patient is referred to hospital because he had been found to have enlarged hilar lymph glands and on further examination, splenomegaly and curious purple lesions on his fingers. His temperature is 101°F. Serum calcium is *3.5 mmol l⁻¹* or 14 mg/100 ml; urinary electrolytes, BUN and phosphorus, and alkaline phosphatase normal. X ray of the hands shows punched out lesions in the metacarpals underlying the purple skin lesions. Serum globulin is 50 g/litre. What is the diagnosis?

Answer 1. Primary hyperparathyroidism. Go on to **4.31**.
2. Metastases. Go on to **4.32**.
3. Sarcoidosis. Go on to **4.33**.

4.28 Your answer—primary hyperparathyroidism.
No. You are guessing, the patient has hypercalcaemia but does not have any of the other evidence of primary hyperparathyroidism such as low serum phosphate, high serum chloride, low TRP. You would have known these facts if you had paid careful attention to what you are reading. Go back and read **4.21** carefully. This is important material that you may not dream through.

4.29 Your answer—secondary hyperparathyroidism.
You are not correct. The history of the excessive milk and alkali intake is an obvious clue to the correct diagnosis and the high serum bicarbonate is confirmation of the true diagnosis. Read **4.24** again and then answer the question.

4.30 You should not be reading this. Follow the instructions.

4.31 Your answer—primary hyperparathyroidism:
You are incorrect. Against primary hyperparathyroidism are the following: normal serum phosphorus and electrolytes. In any case everything leads to an alternative diagnosis. Read **4.24** again, then answer **4.27**.

4.32 Your answer—metastases.
You are guessing. It is true there are punched out lesions in the hands and hypercalcaemia, but there are a host of other findings which are pointers to another diagnosis. Read **4.24** again, but please pay attention to its contents. Then read the question in **4.27** again and answer it correctly.

4.33 Your answer—sarcoidosis.
You are correct. Good. Infantile hypercalcaemia in Britain was common until vitamin D supplements in infant foods were reduced in quan-

tity. It seems likely that most but not all cases of infantile hypercalcaemia were due to vitamin D intoxication. In recovery from acute renal failure caused by rhabdomyolysis, hypercalcaemia has been frequently observed. This often gives rise to the 'red eyes' seen in renal failure with acute rises in the plasma Ca × P product to more than 70 when expressed as mg/100 ml (not SI units). This is a good opportunity to review the symptoms and signs associated with hypercalcaemia. Mild hypercalcaemia usually is asymptomatic i.e. it is a laboratory finding not associated with any symptoms. The most characteristic symptoms of hypercalcaemia are thirst, polyuria and nocturia with dysphagia and lethargy. Sometimes a peculiar metallic taste in the mouth is a leading complaint. The polyuria is due to a reduction in renal concentrating power, with a fall of the maximal osmolality to isosthenuria (i.e. equal to plasma) and then hypotonic urine when nephrogenic diabetes insipidus develops. The urine has an osmolality lower than that of plasma, often in the region of 150 mOsm/kg (remember plasma is usually around 285–290 mOsm/kg). In childhood this lack of concentrating ability may not be noticed in the day, but at night nocturnal enuresis may be a prominent manifestation. In the adult nocturia and thirst are noticeable, but the hypotonic urine does not respond to the administration of vasopressin so that the condition is defined as a nephrogenic form of diabetes insipidus. The suggested mechanism at molecular level is the formation of a tight calcium–ATP complex which is an inhibitor of Na–K–ATPase, the enzyme responsible for sodium transport and important in the generation of renal medullary hyperosmolality of the counter current multiplier. There may be an RTA (renal tubular acidosis) syndrome with impairment of acidification of the urine. Hypercalcuria is present, and hyperpotassuria and hypermagnesuria may also be found. Nephrocalcinosis and renal stone commonly develop in hypercalcaemia, but remember that nephrocalcinosis may be microscopic and only visible on renal biopsy. Look at Fig. 4.33 which shows nephrocalcinosis in distal RTA. Psychiatric disorders are of major importance in the presence of hypercalcaemia, including manic depression. It has been shown to be worthwhile in all patients with psychotic disorders to perform a plasma calcium estimation, and paranoid states, drowsiness and hallucinations are common in patients with serum calcium levels of over 15 mg/100 ml or *3.75 mmol l⁻¹*. Gastrointestinal symptoms include constipation, nausea and vomiting, with dysphagia being occasionally prominent. Pancreatitis may be present in hyperparathyroidism, hypervitaminosis D and carcinomatous hypercalcaemia.

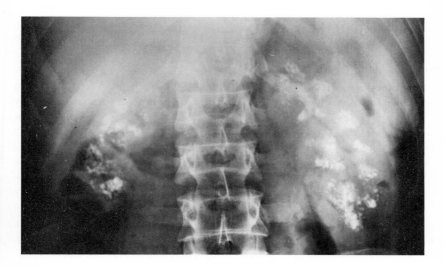

Fig. 4.33a

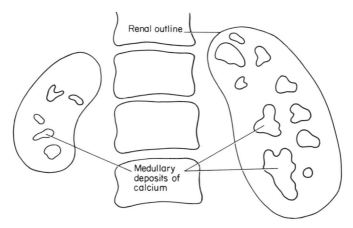

Fig. 4.33b

Question A man suffering from paranoia is found to have a serum calcium of 14 mg/100 ml or *3.5 mmol l⁻¹* in a routine survey. Do you think there is commonly an increased evidence of mental disease in hyper-calcaemic states?

Answer 1. Yes. Go on to **4.35**.
2. No. Go on to **4.34**.

4.34 Your answer—there is no connection.

No. You really are not paying attention. Read **4.33** again. Bear in mind that many patients in psychiatric hospitals have been discovered by routine serum calcium measurements to be suffering from primary hyperparathyroidism. Read **4.33** again.

4.35 Your answer—yes there is a connection.

Correct. Central nervous system depression is frequent with a loss of tendon jerks, hypotonia and loss of visual acuity. Eye changes include red eyes, corneal limbal calcification, and very rarely (particularly in hyperparathyroidism) a band keratopathy where a layer of calcification is formed in the corneal epithelium running across the front of the cornea. Hyperparathyroidism in renal failure gives rise to a high calcium concentration in the skin associated with itching and frequently relieved by parathyroidectomy. Ultraviolet light has also produced good results, and hot baths and saunas are occasionally helpful. Antihistamines are likewise useful. The definitive treatment has yet to be found.

ECG changes in *hypercalcaemia* are as follows: Q-T is short and the Q-T ratio is less than 1. T waves are normal flat or inverted. *In hypocalcaemia* in *contrast* the Q-T interval is prolonged due to an elongated RS-T segment with normal T waves. Remember that in *hypokalaemia* the Q-T interval is elongated but there are *flat and wide T waves*.

Question Look at figure. What is your diagnosis?

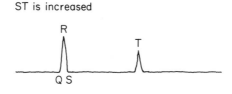

Fig. 4.35

Answer 1. Hypocalcaemia. Go on to **4.37**.
2. Hypercalcaemia. Go on to **4.39**.
3. Hypokalaemia. Go on to **4.41**.

4.36   Your answer—it may not work.

You are partly correct, but only if too small an amount is given. Go back to **4.37** and read it carefully. No point is guessing. It only shows you are not reading properly.

4.37   Your answer—hypocalcaemia.

Good. The treatment of *hypercalcaemia* is aimed at: 1) correcting the state of dehydration consequent on the state nephrogenic diabetes insipidus. 2) Sodium diuresis. This often lowers the serum calcium by 2 mg/100 ml or *0.5 mmol l*$^{-1}$. It should be carried out by giving intravenous furosemide 40 mg with intravenous saline 2—4 litres per day, with a careful watch for signs of neck vein engorgement, shortness of breath, basal crepitations, peripheral oedema and the development of hypertension. It is advantageous to monitor central venous pressure and/or pulmonary wedge pressure. Intravenous sodium bicarbonate may be needed to correct the acidosis in hyperparathyroidism, given in an i.v. dose of 100 mEq daily with more given according to the Pco_2 and pH values. 3) Lowering the plasma calcium level directly. This can be done by:

(a) giving intravenous sodium hydrogen phosphate at a pH of 7.4. The danger of this therapy (which results in complexing of calcium with phosphate, the insoluble calcium phosphate being extracted from the blood and being sequestered in the liver or in the arterial walls) is that it can cause widespread metastatic calcification in a minority of patients.

(b) Steroids should be tried, whatever the cause of the hypercalcaemia, in a dosage of prednisone 60 mg per day. In tumour hypercalcaemia, vitamin D intoxication, sarcoidosis and some cases of hyperparathyroidism this is efficacious in reducing plasma calcium levels.

(c) Giving i.v. EDTA to chelate calcium. Standard atomic absorption flame photometric techniques are not capable of differentiating calcium bound to EDTA from free (and therefore potentially toxic) calcium ion, but there are standard biochemical methods for differentiating ionized from chelated calcium and these should be requested before the blood is sent to the laboratory. Ionized calcium can be estimated, with little difficulty, by a flow-through electrode marketed by Orion, and ionized calcium will be reduced by EDTA therapy even if the total calcium method in use in the hospital laboratory cannot differentiate between the total and EDTA bound calcium.

(d) *Peritoneal dialysis* using a solution free of calcium is temporarily effective in lowering the plasma calcium level, as is haemodialysis using a calcium concentration of 3 mg/100 ml or *0.75 mmol l*$^{-1}$. This is less than the concentration of the normal ionized calcium in plasma, and because the protein bound 50 per cent of plasma calcium is not available for exchange across the dialysis membrane it is necessary to have the maximal chemical gradient across the membrane between the diffusible calcium in the blood and that in the dialysate.

(e) Injection of *salmon calcitonin* has been used to lower plasma calcium levels successfully. However, it is costly material and some people are allergic to the fish protein. I use 100 units (M.R.C.) b.d.

(f) *Infusion of sodium sulphate*: Increase in urinary calcium excretion is brought about by the excretion in the urine of the non-absorbable anion sulphate. This therapy is less effective than phosphate therapy.

(g) *Mithramycin*. Intravenous injection of mithramycin is useful in the therapy of malignant hypercalcaemia; it acts by inhibiting the growth of malignant cells. It is however, toxic to the bone marrow. It should be stressed that therapy of hypercalcaemia is often totally unsatisfactory and may be dangerous. Phosphate infusions may cause metastatic calcification; EDTA may cause haematuria and renal damage. Frusemide, saline and calcitonin are effective.

Question What is the danger of controlling hypercalcaemia with intravenous phosphate?

Answer 1. May not work. Go on to **4.36**.
2. Metastatic calcification. Go on to **4.40**.
3. Hypouricaemia. Go on to **4.38**.

4.38   Your answer—hyperuricaemia.
If you pulled out this as an answer your mind must be pretty short of facts. Do not waste time. Learn carefully. Go back and read **4.37** again.

4.39   Your answer—hypercalcaemia.
No. Q-T is short in hypercalcaemia and long in this case. You have not read **4.35** carefully enough. Quickly read it again. Draw out the various ECG changes in hypocalcaemia, hypokalaemia, and hypercalcaemia, before you try the question again.

4.40   Your answer—metastatic calcification.
You are correct. Hypocalcaemia is a frequent problem. It is defined as a plasma calcium of less than 9 mg/100 ml or *2.25 mmol l^{-1}*. The causes of hypocalcaemia should be differentiated into those due to a fall in plasma albumin concentration alone (i.e. a fall in the protein bound fraction of calcium as a result of any of the numerous causes of hypo-

albuminaemia e.g. malnutrition, nephrotic syndrome, cirrhosis and steatorrhoea) and those due to a fall in total plasma calcium without a fall in plasma albumin level i.e. true hypocalcaemia.

1. Hypoparathyroidism. This condition is most commonly the result of surgery on the thyroid gland where the parathyroids were removed unwittingly in the course of subtotal thyroidectomy, but may be the result of congenital or acquired disease of the parathyroids or follow ^{131}I therapy for thyrotoxicosis. The state of hypoparathyroidism may be obvious within 24 hours after surgery on the thyroid with the development of tingling round the mouth and in fingers and toes accompanied by plasma calcium levels as low as 6 mg/100 ml. On the other hand, it may take special tests of intravenous EDTA infusion to demonstrate an increase in the time needed for restoration of serum calcium to normal from the induced hypocalcaemic levels; this demonstrates a mild functional impairment of the parathyroid glands after thyroid surgery. It has also been demonstrated that there is a decrease in parathyroid hormone levels in patients who have received radio-iodine therapy for hyper-thyroidism. In hypoparathyroidism plasma levels of parathyroid hormone are low or absent in peripheral venous blood and TRP is elevated to 0.90 to 0.95. Surgical hypoparathyroidism, where some parathyroid tissue has been left undamaged, often recovers spontaneously within 2 years, but if not, vitamin D therapy is required: for this purpose 1 α OH vitamin D_3 given in arachis oil, orally in a dose of 2 γ per day, or 1,25 (OH)$_2$ vitamin D_3 in a similar dose is usually adequate to restore plasma calcium levels to normal. In hypoparathyroidism of congenital, idiopathic or acquired (post surgical or post ^{131}Iodine) origin, the biochemical changes are hypocalcaemia, hyperphosphataemia, elevated TRP; urine with little calcium in it.

Question A patient had ^{131}I therapy for thyrotoxicosis 4 years ago. He is asymptomatic. He now has the following biochemical findings:

Plasma calcium = 7 mg/100 ml or *1.75 mmol l^{-1}*.
Plasma inorganic phosphorus = 8 mg/100 ml or *2.6 mmol l^{-1}*.
TRP = 0.95.
What is the diagnosis?

Answer 1. Hypothyroidism. Go on to **4.42**.
        2. Hypoparathyroidism. Go on to **4.44**.

4.41   Your answer—hypokalaemia.

Well you are half right, half wrong. There is a prolonged Q-T in the ECG but also flat and wide T waves in hypokalaemia. These are not present in the figure in the question. So go back and read **4.35** again. This time do so carefully.

4.42   Your answer—the diagnosis is hypothyroidism.

No. The patient may have hypothyroidism but you have been given no biochemical evidence for this. Therefore you cannot make the diagnosis. Now go back and read **4.40** again.

4.43   Your   answer—pseudohypoparathyroidism.   You   are   correct. Let us now go on to:

2. Hypocalcaemia in vitamin D lack. Hypocalcaemia is common in rickets in childhood or osteomalacia in the adult, whether simply due to dietary vitamin D deficiency, difficulty in vitamin D absorption in steatorrhoea, or due to vitamin D resistance as in renal failure where 1,25 dehydroxy vitamin D_3 is not formed from 25 hydroxycholecalciferol due to absence of 1 hydroxylase enzyme which is only present in the kidney. In renal failure uncalcified osteoid is frequently present and serum calcium levels are lower than normal. We have described rapidly maturing cataracts in patients with severe hypocalcaemia associated with osteomalacia and renal failure, with intractable serum calcium levels of 4 to 6 mg/100 ml being responsible for the development of a cataract of metabolic origin similar to the cataracts seen in the hypocalcaemia of hypoparathyroidism. Since the description of these cases 1 α hydroxycholecalciferol and 1,25 $(OH)_2$ D_3 have been introduced commercially, and with an oral dose of 2 to 10 γ per day, together with an oral calcium supplement of 1 g/day it is now easy to treat low serum calcium levels and elevate them to normal. In the hypocalcaemia of nutritional osteomalacia (adult rickets) there is normally an elevated alkaline phosphatase and also a normal plasma inorganic phosphorus level.

3. Neonatal hypocalcaemia. Every practising nephrologist sees severe hypocalcaemia in neonates given cow's milk i.e. a very high phosphate diet, which causes a high plasma inorganic phosphorus level and a depressed serum calcium with tetany and convulsions. A typical biochemical profile is:

plasma calcium   7 mg/100 ml or *1.75 mmol l^{-1}*.
plasma inorganic phosphorus   8 mg/100 ml, or *2.6 mmol l^{-1}*.

The condition rapidly responds to withdrawal of cow's milk and substitution of an appropriate 'humanized' formula. The surprising fact is that despite the vast number of neonates fed on untreated cow's milk only a very small proportion develop tetany. It is likely that there is a temporary depression of parathyroid gland function in the first few weeks of life, as a result of the increased PTH levels in the mother, and the very high plasma calcium levels in the neonate at birth and that these contribute to the hypocalcaemia by inhibiting the parathyroid gland before and after birth.

4. Hypocalcaemia in malignant disease. Adrenalectomy in patients with widespread bony metastases of carcinoma of the breast may be associated with hypocalcaemia due to bone reconstitution acting as a sponge for the circulating calcium. However, paradoxical hypocalcaemia can be seen from time to time with osteoblastic metastases of carcinoma of bronchus, breast and prostate, presumably due to the metastases acting as a sponge and sucking up the calcium to form new bone. Medullary carcinoma of the thyroid is associated with high plasma levels of calcitonin and sometimes there is associated hypocalcaemia. Remember that salmon calcitonin is used as a therapy for hypercalcaemia.

5. Acute pancreatitis. In acute pancreatitis calcium soaps are formed throughout the mesenteric fat and this removal of calcium is probably quite adequate to cause a fall of plasma calcium levels. It is worthwhile remembering that ionized calcium in the ECF is 15×50 mg $=$ 750 mg totally (*18.75 mmol*), so that it is rather remarkable that the plasma calcium level falls only to 6 mg/100 ml (*1.25 mmol l^{-1}*) or thereabouts due to its constant replenishment by destruction of bone stores of calcium. There is a suggestion that in acute pancreatitis hypocalcaemia may result from high glucagon levels stimulating calcitonin secretion.

In *osteopetrosis* there may be a low plasma calcium level because of the high levels of circulating calcitonin. In *magnesium deficiency* there is a resistance to action of vitamin D and to PTH and resultant hypocalcaemia; administration of magnesium to repair the magnesium deficit causes sensitivity to vitamin D to be restored and so correction of the hypocalcaemia results.

Question In a patient suffering from chronic alcoholism the following biochemical results are found.

1. Serum calcium 5.0 mg/100 ml or *1.25 mmol* l^{-1}.
2. Serum inorganic phosphorus 2.0 mg/100 ml or *0.7 mmol* l^{-1}.
3. Serum magnesium 0.8 mg/100 ml or *0.3 mmol* l^{-1}.

Will vitamin D therapy alone bring about an increase in serum calcium level?

Answer 1. Yes. Go on to **4.46**.
2. No. Go on to **4.48**.

4.44 Your answer—hypoparathyroidism.

You are correct. Good. Now in patients with idiopathic (non-surgical) hypoparathyroidism there is a concomitant association of typical nail changes (due to monilia of the nails), and vaginal and oral moniliasis may be present. There is also an increase in the incidence of Addison's disease. Congestive heart failure and papilloedema may be features of idiopathic hypoparathyroidism. In children idiopathic hypothyroidism may cause growth retardation and result eventually in dwarfism if untreated. Cataracts are common in hypoparathyrodism. X-ray changes in hypoparathyroidism are calcification of the basal ganglia; subcutaneous calcification is never found in hypoparathyroidism. There is, however, a condition known as pseudohypoparathyroidism, an X linked recessive disorder seen in twice as many females as in males, in whom there is end organ unresponsiveness to circulating PTH which is present in normal or increased amount in the plasma and in whom, after PTH injection, the normal increase in urinary cyclic AMP is not seen. This suggests that the receptors for PTH in the cells do not respond in a normal manner to the PTH secreted. Plasma calcium level in this disease may be low or normal, changing cyclically for reasons unknown. Clinically there is a characteristic picture: flat faced, short and obese, the female: male ratio 2:1. Brachydactyly is present because of premature closure of the metacarpal and metatarsal epiphyses. This mainly affects the first, fourth and fifth metacarpals and gives rise to a dimple over the metacarpal heads when the fist is clenched. This is known as Albright's sign. Hypertension, mental defect, diabetes mellitus and hypothyroidism are common. Cataracts, subcutaneous calcification and calcification of the basal ganglia are common in this disease, but subcutaneous calcification *does not* occur in true hypoparathyroidism: its presence is suggestive of pseudohypoparathyroidism. The diagnosis is best made by giving 600 units of 'Parathormone' preparation intramuscularly every 8 hours for 2 days. In true hypoparathyroidism there is at least a doubling of the 24 hour phosphorus excretion in the urine, when compared with control values. In pseudo-hypoparathyroidism there is end-organ refractoriness to parathyroid hormone and thus there is little or no phosphaturic response to 'Parathormone' infusion. Remember that 'Parathormone' is a proprietary name of a parathyroid extract, and is *not* synonymous with parathyroid hormone.

Question A female 18 year old patient is found to have cataracts and a serum calcium of 7 mg/100 ml (*1.75 mmol l*$^{-1}$), a serum inorganic P of 8 mg/100 ml (*2.6 mmol l*$^{-1}$), BUN 18 mg/100 ml (*3 mmol l*$^{-1}$). X ray of the skull shows basal ganglia calcification. She has subcutaneous calcification in the hands. 600 units of parathyroid extract, 1 ml 8 hourly for 2 days gives no increase in phosphaturia. What is the diagnosis?

Answer 1. Hypoparathyroidism. Go on to **4.45**.
2. Pseudohypoparathyroidism. Go on to **4.43**.

4.45 Your answer—hypoparathyroidism.
In true hypoparathyroidism there is no subcutaneous calcification, and also there is a doubling of the phosphate excretion in the urine after appropriate parathyroid extract. These facts were quite clearly stated in **4.44**. The lack of immediate recall is suggestive of your not having memorized these points. Kindly read **4.44** again, and answer the question without guessing.

4.46 Your answer—yes.
This is not so. In the presence of severe hypomagnesaemia there is resistance to the hypercalcaemic action of vitamin D. This is clearly stated in **4.43**. You have missed it by not reading carefully. Now read **4.43** again and then you will get the correct answer without guesswork.

4.47 Your answer—Chvostek's sign is abnormal.
Unfortunately you are guessing. Chvostek's sign in the upper lip is seen only in 1/3 of normal people. This is clearly stated in **4.48**, so you need to read it again; you have probably missed other important information.

4.48 Your answer—no.
You are correct. Let us now deal with clinical features of hypocalcaemia. Clinical features of hypocalcaemia are striking. They will be dealt with in groups:

1. Neuromuscular. In this section tetany is the overall condition which is divisible into several manifestations of increasing severity.

(a) Paraesthesia-perioral, lingual and in the hands and feet;

(b) Muscle spasms in (1) hands-giving rise to the main d'accoucheur—the male midwife's hand—look at the photograph and then the reason for the name becomes obvious.

(2) Feet giving rise to painful spasms. In both hands and feet the patient is unable voluntarily to oppose the spasm.

(c) Laryngeal stridor from spasm of the laryngeal muscles.

(d) Spasms of jaw muscles giving rise to difficulties in deglutition and speech.

(e) full scale convulsions with loss of consciousness.

The physical signs of tetany are as follows:

I. Trousseau's sign. A blood pressure cuff is placed on the arm and inflated for 3 minutes at a pressure above systolic: in 2/3 of patients with latent tetany Trousseau's test precipitates overt tetany in the hand on the occluded side.

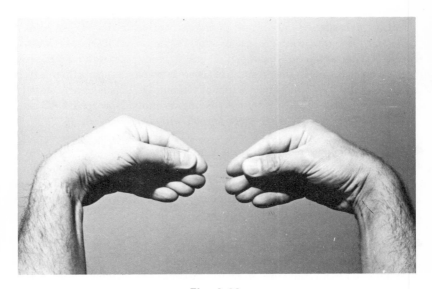

Fig. 4.46

II. Chvostek's sign. If the facial nerve is tapped as it emerges anterior to the lower half of the external ear there is a reflex contraction of the facial muscles of the side of the mouth, the ala nasi and the orbicularis oculi muscles. The response in which only the upper lip muscles twitch is found in about 1/3 of normal persons, but if eyelids and ala nasi are involved this is commonly indicative of latent tetany.

The next stage of tetany is that of tetanic convulsions. These are generalized grand mal epileptiform convulsions, and are associated with loss of consciousness, tonic and clonic phases, tongue biting and incontinence.

Ocular changes: the development of cataract is important in severe hypocalcaemia of any cause. It is not only important to think of this in the differential diagnosis of cataract, but also important to prevent its development by appropriate therapy of hypocalcaemia.

Dermatologic disorders: Moniliasis of the nails and skin is found in many patients with persistent hypocalcaemia and idiopathic hypoparathyroidism. The teeth are usually hypoplastic and tend to fall out early. Eczema is a common problem.

Mental changes: Dementia, psychoses and confusion are frequently found in hypocalcaemia. It is therefore worthwhile to perform plasma calcium determination in psychotics. They may be associated with calcification of the basal ganglia, frontal lobe, and dentate nucleus.

Question Chvostek's sign is found over the upper lip only in an otherwise normal person. Is this necessarily abnormal?

Answer 1. Yes. Go on to **4.47**.
2. No. Go on to **4.50**.

4.49 Your answer—10 mg.

You are guessing. Either you remember or you don't. Go back and learn **4.50**. This is a meaningful learning experience not a day-dreaming exercise.

4.50 Your answer—no.

Chvostek's sign in the upper lip occurs in 1/3 normal people. Good. What causes of tetany are there other than hypocalcaemia? The following cause tetany, apart from hypocalcaemia:

(1) Overbreathing—commonly found in hysterical young women. This is the commonest cause of tetany seen in the hospital emergency room. It is associated with a severe alkalosis and a low $P\text{co}_2$. Look at a typical example of blood gas findings.

$$pH = 7.55.$$
$$P\text{co}_2 = 20 \text{ mm.}$$
$$P\text{co}_2 = 85 \text{ mm.}$$

The reason for the tetany is a reduction in the plasma ionized calcium level consequent upon the alkalosis, so that plasma ionized calcium may fall from *1.25 to 0.75 mmol l^{-1}*. (5.0 mg/100 ml to 3.0 mg/100 ml) although total plasma calcium level may be unchanged.

(2) Hypokalaemia. The hypokalaemic patient will develop tetany when plasma K level is below 2.5 mEq/l.

(3) Hypomagnesaemia. A fall of plasma magnesium to *0.4 mmol l^{-1}* (1 mg/100 ml) or less may cause tetany.

(4) Metabolic alkalosis: inhibition of excessive sodium bicarbonate can cause clinical tetany when there is a rise of the plasma pH, by the same mechanism as is found in respiratory alkalosis. *The treatment of tetany* is to treat the primary condition causing it:

(1) Hypocalcaemia. Therapy of hypocalcaemia is (a) *short term*: intravenous injection slowly over a period of 5 minutes of 10 ml of 10 per cent calcium gluconate, (this contains 90 mg of elemental calcium. Remember never give anything quickly i.v. (other than Diazoxide) because a high concentration may reach the myocardium or the medulla with fatal results. 1 g of calcium gluconate contains 90 mg of calcium but calcium chloride (10 per cent) is cheaper, and 10 ml of this contains 360 mg of elemental calcium, but may cause necrosis if it gets outside the vein. (b) *Long term:* Solve the cause of the hypocalcaemia. In hypoparathyroidism giving vitamin D in one of its forms such as 1,25 $(OH)_2 D_3$ or 1α OH vitamin D_3 or 1,25 $(OH)_2 D_3$ 2–10) γ/day orally, with if necessary oral calcium supplements—0.5 to 1 g/day may suffice. It may be necessary to give magnesium supplements if the hypocalcaemia is found to be resistant to adequate dosage of 1α OH vitamin D_3 or 1,25 $(OH)_2 D_3$. In chronic renal failure depression of the elevated plasma inorganic phosphorus levels by means of phosphate binders such as aluminium hydroxide may result in restoration of plasma calcium levels to normal. Addition of oral calcium loads in massive dosage of up to 20 g/day as calcium lactate must be regarded with a degree of caution because of the possibility of metastatic calcification.

Question How much elemental calcium is there in 1 g of calcium gluconate?

Answer 1. 10 mg. Go on to **4.49**.
2. 90 mg. Go on to **4.53**.
3. 360 mg. Go on to **4.51**.

4.51   Your answer—360 mg.
You have guessed the wrong answer. You have confused calcium chloride with calcium gluconate. Please read **4.50** again. Learn it with greater care this time.

4.52   Your answer—absorptive hypercalciuria.
It is clearly stated that urinary calcium did not rise after an oral calcium load. Read **4.57** again. The material is not easy but Dr. Pak's classification is currently the state of the art, and you must know it.

4.53   Your answer—90 mg of elemental calcium.
You are correct. Most of the calcium in the body is in the skeleton. The skeleton is quite remarkable. It consists of a collagen meshwork in which the calcium salts are laid down. Let us have a look at the collagen. The collagen is made from submicroscopic fibres of tropocollagen, which are so spaced that nucleation of calcium-containing salts can occur between the ends of the tropocollagen fibres. Thus the calcium salt crystals are laid down and orientated by the collagen fibres. The tropocollagen fibres are made of chains of tripeptides in which one of the 3 amino acids is glycine. Thus collagen consists of a triple helix of these chains each of which is built up of tripeptide units.

The salts of which the skeleton is formed consists of hydroxyapatite $Ca_{10} (PO_4)_6 (OH)_2$ and amorphous calcium phosphate. At present it is thought that amorphous calcium phosphate is first laid down in the interfibre zone between the tropocollagen bundles and that much of it later changes to hydroxyapatite. Hydroxyapatite is not a simple compound, for in the bony crystal is incorporated some carbonate and also quantities of other ions such as magnesium, sodium and potassium. The skeleton may contain appreciable amounts of fluoride, which may alter the crystal characteristics totally.

In hydroxyapatite there can be replacement of phosphate by carbonate ion at the crystal surface, and in the acidosis of chronic renal failure this bicarbonate is titrated off to buffer the 30–50 mEq of protons liberated metabolically each day and where excretion is impaired. Also at the surface of the crystal lattice are the ions, sodium, magnesium, fluoride and potassium. Lead, radium and plutonium are heavy metals taken up by bone in the crystal lattice in the case of poisoning. This in the case of the long half like radio-isotopes radium and plutonium, which are bone seeking, and thus may cause osteogenic sarcoma.

The mature skeleton consists of 65—70 per cent by weight of calcium phosphate salts, the remainder being organic material, 95 per cent of which is collagen; 1/3 of the collagen is glycine, you will recall from the structure of tropocollagen. Hydroxyproline accounts for about 14 per cent of the amino acid content of collagen. It is formed *in situ* by hydroxylation of proline. The destruction of bone liberates hydroxyproline, which is not reused in the body and this is excreted in the urine in free or 'bound' forms in which it is a constituent of peptides. Hydroxyproline excretion is a useful marker of bone catabolism (like 3 methylhistidine is a marker for muscle catabolism). It is fairly easy to measure on an AutoAnalyser without recourse to a sophisticated amino acid analyser. As collagen matures there develop biochemical ionic linkages within the tropocollagen subunits and between the collagen polypeptide chains. According to Avioli PTH causes an acceleration of the normal maturation of bone, but the subject is still in the early stages of investigation and as yet only partly understood.

Question Is hydroxyproline reutilized by the body?

Answer 1. Yes. Go on to **4.55**.
         2. No. Go on to **4.57**.

4.54 Your answer—hypercalciuria of renal tubular origin.
Correct.

Hypercalcaemia in malignancy. Some solid tumours cause hypercalcaemia without iPTH levels being elevated in the plasma. In a group of these tumours with normal iPTH it has been shown that the tumour produces increased amounts of the prostaglandin PGE_2 which causes bone absorption. The prostaglandin synthetase inhibitor, Indomethacin, causes a fall in plasma calcium levels in these patients pari passu with a fall in plasma $iPGE_2$ levels: aspirin, also an inhibitor of prostaglandin synthesis, has the same effect. In multiple myeloma the plasma $iPGE_2$ levels are normal but there seems to be a direct stimulation of osteoclasis by a substance produced by the myeloma cells. Corticosteroids may act in some tumour hypercalcaemias by their inhibition of synthesis of prosta-glandins. Let us go over some of the physiology of calcium again on the principle that the more mud you throw at a wall, the more sticks.

The physiologic action of calcium at cellular level is:

(1) To control the permeability of the cell surface which has calcium actually located in the surface itself.

(2) To maintain intracellular cytoplasmic ionized calcium levels.

(3) To control initiation and propogation of action potentials.

(4) Initiate muscular contraction by an ATP dependent movement to calcium actomysin.

(5) Response to action potentials is often dependent on the presence of calcium before acetylcholine can be released: thus secretion of adrenal cortical and medullary hormones, anterior and posterior pituitary hor-mones and insulin and glucagon secretion are all dependent on the presence of calcium.

(6) Calcium dependent ATPase is found in muscle.

(7) Calcium can be taken up by mitochondria by an energy con-suming process coupled usually but not necessarily, with phosphate accumulation. Release from mitochondria of calcium is caused by PTH and vitamin D.

When PTH is injected i.v. it releases from the kidneys cAMP—the second messenger. How PTH causes bone breakdown is not fully under-stood—it appears to first cause release of calcium from the bone and then collagen breakdown products appear; the most readily characterized is hydroxyproline which is excreted without change in the urine. Control of parathyroid secretion is mediated by plasma ionized calcium and magnesium level by a feedback system which is remarkably efficient. A fall in plasma ionized calcium levels stimulate parathyroid hormone (PTH) secretion. Similarly PTH secretion is stimulated by low plasma magnesium levels. In the presence of elevated plasma ionized calcium or magnesium levels PTH secretion is inhibited. Parathyroid hormone is one of the major factors in plasma calcium homeostasis by means of a feedback mechanism. It is the hormone responsible for the metabo-lism of bone and thus is essential in the normal processes of remodel-ling of the skeleton, of wear and tear, and of growth. The second hormone of uncertain importance in man, but of great importance in lower animals is calcitonin, secreted by the thyroid C cells, and res-ponsible for anabolism of bone and lowering of the plasma calcium level. Calcitonin is secreted in increased amounts in response to an elevation of the plasma calcium levels and in response to increased plasma gastrin levels. Growth hormone, testosterone and oestrogen are all anabolic hormones which cause the build-up of bone. Thyroid hormone increases the catabolism of bone, as do adrenal steroids.

Now let us examine what you have retained in this chapter. Look at the 3 statements and choose the correct answer:

Statement 1. Renal failure is associated with low levels of 1,25 $(OH)_2$ D_3.

Statement 2. Urinary calcium is normally more than 350 mg/day in a woman.

Statement 3. 50—70 per cent of the filtered calcium is reabsorbed in the proximal tubule.

Answer 1. All statement are true. Go on to **4.58**.
   2. All statements are false. Go on to **4.59**.
   3. Statement 1 is true, 2 and 3 false. Go on to **4.60**.
   4. Statement 2 is true, 1 and 3 false. Go on to **4.61**.
   5. Statement 3 is true, 2 and 3 false. Go on to **4.62**.
   6. Statement 1 and 2 are true, 3 false. Go on to **4.63**.
   7. Statement 1 and 3 are true, 2 false. Go on to **4.64**.
   8. Statement 2 and 3 are true, 1 false. Go on to **4.65**.

4.55 Your answer—yes.

Hydroxyproline is reutilized by the body. You have missed the point. It is not reutilized by the body, so it appears in the urine and the amount excreted is related to bone breakdown. Read **4.53** again.

4.56 Your answer—primary hyperparathyroidism.

It is possible that some of these cases have secondary hyperparathyroidism, but primary does not present like this very often. Read **4.57** so that Pak's classification is fixed in your mind.

4.57 Your answer—hydroxyproline is not reutilized by the body.

Correct. Urinary calcium levels are high when hypercalcaemia is present, unless the patient has renal failure concomitantly. Thus urinary calcium levels are high in idiopathic hypercalcaemia, hyperparathyroidism, and any other cause of hypercalcaemia. Loss of magnesium or sodium in the urine in large quantities may be paralleled by an increase in urine calcium.

Idiopathic hypercalcuria may be conveniently divided into 3 groups, according to Pak's classification.

1) Hyperparathyroidism which is occult, where there is an elevated

PTH level due to primary hyperparathyroidism and a high cAMP concentration in the urine not suppressed by an oral calcium load.

2) Absorptive hypercalcuria where there is an intestinal defect allowing excess calcium absorption from the small bowel resulting in post prandial hypercalcaemia and hypercalcuria. In the fasting state urine calcium excreted is not increased.

3) Idiopathic hypercalcuria of renal tubular origin has the following characteristics: normal plasma calcium, high urinary calcium, high fasting urinary cAMP and a normal urinary cAMP after an oral calcium load. It is possible, but not proven, that in these patients there is a state of secondary hyperparathyroidism.

Now let us look at an example:

Question A man with recurrent renal stones has a plasma calcium level of 2.5 $mmol$ l^{-1} or 10 mg/100 ml, which does not rise after an oral calcium load, a urinary 24 hour calcium excretion of 8.75 $mmol$ or 350 mg/day and a fasting urinary cAMP which is high. What condition is present here?

Answer 1. Absorptive hypercalciuria. Go on to **4.52**.
2. Idiopathic hypercalcaemia of renal tubular origin. Go on to **4.54**.
3. Primary hyperparathyroidism. Go on to **4.56**.

4.58 Your answer—all statements are true.
No. You have not read the material on the normal amount of calcium in the urine. Go back to **4.1** again and read on until you have discovered the error.

4.59 Your answer—all statements are false.
You are guessing about statements 1 and 3. Start again at **4.1**.

4.60 Your answer—statement 3 is correct.
You should read the section on renal physiology again. Then choose the correct answer.

4.62 Your answer—statement 3 is true.
Well that is correct, but 1 is also correct. You should read the section on vitamin D metabolism again.

4.63 Your answer—statement 3 is false.
No you have forgotten most of the chapter. Look through it again.

4.64   Your answer—statements 1 and 3 are true.

You are correct. Before going on to Chapter 4 you might want to look up some important articles and books.

The monograph by Nordin; Calcium, Magnesium and Phosphate Metabolism is particularly good.

Schrier R. *Renal and Electrolyte Disorders.* Little Brown, Boston.

Articles by:

(1) Ritz E. *Contributions to Nephrology* S. Karger, Basel. *Vol*

(2) DeLuca H. (1978) in *Advances in Experimental Biology and Medicine 103 Vitamin D Metabolism.* Massry Ritz Rapado (Ed.) Plenum Press, New York.

Are highly recommended.

Tashjian A. H. (1975) Prostaglandin hypercalcaemia and cancer. *New Engl. J. Med.* **293**, 1317–13.

4.65   Your answer—1 is false.

No. 1 is true, 2 is false. You have remembered little of the chapter. Start it again and learn it more carefully.

Chapter 5
Magnesium

5.1 Magnesium is the cinderella of the divalent ions. It is ubiquitous in the body. Its presence is necessary for the action of numerous enzymes, yet remarkably little is known about its physiology. Part of the reason for the lack of knowledge when compared, for instance, to calcium, is that there is no electrode readily available for measuring magnesium ion, and that the radio-isotopes of magnesium have a short half life and a relatively low specific activity so limiting their usefulness to research workers. However, you must have a good idea of what is known. Magnesium is principally an intracellular cation about 1000 mEq being found inside the cells and another 1000 mEq being in the bone crystals. Extracellular fluid magnesium is in a low concentration, in the plasma the concentration is between *0.75 and 1 mmol l^{-1}* or 1.5 and 2.0 mEq/litre but varies considerably. Remember *0.5 mmol = 24 mg of magnesium.* 1 mEq = 12 mg of magnesium. The mechanisms for maintaining a constant plasma concentration are less efficient than those for calcium although often sharing common mechanisms. Also variations in plasma magnesium of 6-fold from *0.5 to 3 mmol l^{-1}* (1 to 6 mEq/litre) may not be fatal, unlike plasma calcium variations which differ much less in health and disease i.e. only about 3 fold *1.25−3.75 mmol l^{-1}* (5−15 mg/100 ml). Magnesium is however, apart from about *6.25 mmol* (150 mg) in the ECF, principally an intracellular cation. Protein bound magnesium is found in proportions varying from 20 to 30 per cent, the rest being diffusible and mostly ionized. The total body content of magnesium is about 2000 mEq or *1000 mmol.* Half of this (1000 mEq or *500 mmol*) is found in bone in the crystal lattice and 1000 mEq or *500 mmol* is found in the intracellular compartment. In renal disease more Mg is held in the bone crystal lattice than in normals. You remember that 1 per cent is found in the ECF, and of that in the plasma 20−30 per cent is found to be protein bound. The remainder is diffusible and mostly ionized, but some is non-ionized diffusible magnesium, being chelated by citrate and other organic acids.

Question How much magnesium is in the intracellular compartment?

Answer 1. 100 mEq (*50 mmol*). Go on to **5.3**.

2. 1000 mEq (*500 mmol*). Go on to **5.5**.
3. 10 mEq (*5 mmol*). Go on to **5.6**.

5.2   Your answer—all of it.
   You are incorrect. The exchangeable magnesium is not identical with total body magnesium. You have not read **5.6** carefully. Read it again.

5.3   Your answer— 100 mEq (*50 mmol*).
   This is a guesswork answer. It is also a bad guess and tells me that if you are not able to concentrate at the beginning of the chapter, then you must either give up learning now and come back to it when you are less tired, or you should forthwith shut out the distractions and start **5.1** again.

5.4   Your answer—1/3 is exchangeable.
   You are correct. Good.

Muscle magnesium: 20 per cent of the total body magnesium is in the muscle. It is the second highest cation in concentration (76 mEq/kg fat free dry weight). Muscle magnesium is frequently measured as a research project although there is little practical application, because the red cell magnesium content gives an indication of cellular magnesium levels without recourse to muscle biopsy. Young erythrocytes contain more magnesium than old cells. Reticulocytes contain up to 50 per cent more magnesium than mature erythrocytes. This is of importance when reviewing data on magnesium content of RBC's in haemolytic anaemias. Normal bone calcium/magnesium ratio is 50 to 1, 60 per cent of the total body magnesium being present in bone. Of this 1/3 is exchangeable and presumably on the surface of the bone crystal-lattice. Magnesium in the diet is found in green vegetables (chlorophyll contains magnesium), cereals, meats, seafood and coconuts. It is difficult on any normal diet to get a low magnesium intake. The minimum needed to be sure to be in positive balance is 3.6 mg (0.3 mEq)/kg body weight/day or *0.15 mmol/ kg day*$^{-1}$ i.e. 21 mEq or *10.5 mmol* for a 70 kg man.
   In magnesium deficiency with a normal bowel 3/4 of dietary magnesium is absorbed from the gut. With high magnesium intake, only 1/4 may be absorbed.

Question How much of the total body magnesium is found in muscle?

Answer 1. 50 per cent. Go on to **5.7**.
          2. 10 per cent. Go on to **5.9**.
          3. 20 per cent. Go on to **5.11**.

5.5 Your answer—1000 mEq.

You are correct. Total body magnesium studies are rendered difficult by the lack of a suitable isotope. In practice only one isotope is available. ^{28}Mg, that has a half life of about 21 hours. This is somewhat difficult to obtain, but with ^{28}Mg, exchangeable magnesium can be measured if the specific activity is high enough to furnish enough radio-activity to count accurately without loading the body with large amounts of stable magnesium. Read this last sentence again, and bear in mind that specific activity is really the concentration of radioactive magnesium in non-radio-active stable magnesium, i.e. μC of ^{28}Mg/mEq of stable magnesium. There is also a very short half life isotope of magnesium, ^{27}Mg, which has a half life of 9.5 minutes. This is only useful for very short experiments and certainly useless as far as measuring Mg_E (exchangeable magnesium) Only 1/3 of the total body magnesium is exchangeable. Thus magnesium research has lagged behind sodium and potassium. Also only in the past 15 years has there been readily available a method which is accurate to measure stable magnesium i.e. atomic absorption spectrophotometry. These are the reasons for the fact that less is known about magnesium than other common cations. Total body magnesium and organ magnesium are measured by direct measurement after acid digestion of the body or the organ.

Question How much of the total body magnesium is exchangeable?

Answer 1. All of it. Go on to **5.2**.
          2. 1/3. Go on to **5.4**.
          3. 2/3. Go on to **5.8**.

5.6 Your answer—10 mEq or *5 mmol.*

This is a really poor guess and, if this is a sign of your present concentration then either stop working now or get out of the distracting interferences. When you can concentrate in peace, start at **5.1** again.

5.7 Your answer—50 per cent of the magnesium is in muscle.

You are not correct. In **5.4** it is clearly stated that 20 per cent of the magnesium is in muscle. You should have remembered that. Read **5.4** again.

5.8   Your answer—2/3 is exchangeable.

You are incorrect. Only 1/3 is exchangeable, the other 2/3 being bound and not available for exchange. Read **5.6** again in case you have missed something else important.

5.9   Your answer—10 per cent.

You are guessing. More than 10 per cent of body magnesium is found in muscle. You should read **5.4** more carefully.

5.10   Your answer—old cells have more magnesium.

No. Your recall is faulty. Read **5.4** again, then answer this question in **5.11** correctly.

5.11   Your answer—20 per cent of body magnesium is found in muscle. Good. You are correct. Now answer the next question:

Question Which contains more magnesium per cell—old cells or reticulocytes?

Answer   1. Old cells. Go on to **5.10**.
          2. Reticulocytes. Go on to **5.12**.
          3. Equal. Go on to **5.13**.

5.12   Your answer—Reticulocytes.

Good. You are correct. The diet of a North European contains about 20 to 40 mEq/day. Of this 30–60 per cent is absorbed and 40–70 per cent is excreted in the faeces. Magnesium continues to be absorbed in renal failure (unlike calcium which is little absorbed from the gut in renal failure). This causes increased plasma levels of magnesium and increased bone stores in renal failure.

In renal failure the lack of impairment of absorption of magnesium suggests that 1,25 $(OH)_2 D_3$ is not essential for the absorption of magnesium from the small intestine. You remember that intestinal calcium absorption is impaired in renal disease because of the necessity of the presence of 1,25 hydroxycholecalciferol to stimulate the formation of mRNA in the intestinal mucosa: the mRNA is responsible for the formation of calcium-binding protein in the intestinal mucosa necessary for calcium absorption. In kidney failure 1,25 dehydroxycholecalciferol cannot be made because of the absence of 1 hydroxylase which converts 25 hydroxycholecalciferol to 1,25 dihydroxycholecalciferol in the kidney.

Question In renal failure is magnesium absorption from the gut seriously impaired?

Answer 1. No. Go on to **5.14**.
         2. Yes. Go on to **5.16**.

5.13   Your answer—they are equal.

That is a reasonable guess, but it is wrong. Read **5.4** again and answer the question in **5.11** correctly. Get yourself away from the distractions and learn properly.

5.14   Your answer—magnesium absorption is not impaired seriously in renal failure.

You are correct. Good. In assessment of magnesium depletion, knowledge of plasma magnesium levels in man is but a poor substitute for knowledge of the body stores of magnesium. Plasma magnesium levels may fall without serious reduction in total body magnesium. Control of magnesium levels in the blood is partially understood. Magnesium is absorbed in the small intestine and excreted by the kidneys. About 25 per cent is absorbed in the proximal tubule and about 70–80 per cent in the ascending loop of Henle, the remainder being absorbed more distally. There is evidence in some species of magnesium secretion, when magnesium loading is performed, but this is in the most distal portions of the nephron. High magnesium levels in the plasma suppress the release of PTH from the parathyroid gland; but secretion of parathyroid hormone stimulated by low magnesium levels is an inefficient feedback system and does not succeed adequately in restoring the levels of plasma magnesium to normal; this is because the amount of magnesium liberated from bone is not adequate to replenish losses, there being relatively little magnesium liberated by PTH from bone when compared to the amount of calcium liberated from the same quantity of bone, remember the bone Ca/Mg ratio is 50 : 1. Also hypomagnesaemia in man may result in bone and intestine becoming resistant to PTH and vitamin D and this may lead to hypocalcaemia which responds not to PTH or vitamin D, but to magnesium. Commonly there is an associated hypokalaemia, possibly a result of hyperaldosteronism induced by contraction of the ECF volume.

Question A man has a serum magnesium of 0.5 mg/100 ml (*0.2 mmol l*$^{-1}$) a serum calcium of *1.25 mmol l*$^{-1}$ or 5.0 mg/100 ml and a serum inorganic phosphate of *1.3 mmol l*$^{-1}$ or 4.0 mg/100 ml. The patient is given

1,25 $(OH)_2$ D_3 but the serum calcium remains *1.25 mmol l^{-1} 5.0 mg/100* ml. What therapy would you advise?

Answer   1. More vitamin D. Go on to **5.15**.
              2. Phosphate. Go on to **5.17**.
              3. Magnesium. Go on to **5.19**.

5.15   Your answer—give more vitamin D.
           This will hardly help. You have not read **5.14** carefully.

5.16   Your answer—magnesium absorption is seriously impaired in renal failure.
           No—this is a guess. You must learn facts and then cogitate upon them. As it is, you are day-dreaming. Read **5.12** carefully again.

5.17   Your answer—give phosphate.
           This is a remarkable guess. The data show normal phosphate levels, so why give phosphate? Read **5.14**.

5.18   Your answer—serum magnesium level will be normal.
           It may be normal but you were asked the question because you should have remembered that serum magnesium levels may be low in hyper-calcaemia of any cause. Go back and read **5.19** again, this time carefully so as to be sure not to have missed some important fact which may be quite vital in the case of patient with electrolyte abnormalities.

5.19   Your answer—magnesium should be given.
           You are correct. Magnesium loss in the urine is increased during diuretic therapy with Edecryn®, Lasix® (furosemide) thiazides and mercurials. This may be of importance because magnesium deficiency, like potassium deficiency, sensitizes the patient to the toxic actions of digitalis glycosides which themselves reduce tubular reabsorption of magnesium. In hypercalcaemia of any cause hypomagnesaemia may be found. Factors influencing tubular reabsorption are shown in Table 5.19. Hyperthyroidism is associated with elevated urinary magnesium excretion and lowered plasma magnesium levels. Primary aldosteronism increases urinary and faecal magnesium excretion so that a severe magnesium deficiency and hypomagnesaemia develops. Calcium binders in the intestine such as phytate and cellulose phosphate, or ion exchange

Table 5.19 Factors affecting tubular reabsorption of magnesium (*after Massry*)

A. Decrease tubular reabsorption
  1. Extracellular fluid volume expansion
  2. Renal vasodilatation
  3. Osmotic diuresis
  4. Diuretic agents
  5. Cardiac glycosides
  6. Hypercalcaemia
  7. Alcohol ingestion
  8. High sodium intake
  9. Growth hormone
 10. Thyroid hormone
 11. Calcitonin
 12. Chronic mineralocorticoid effect
 13. Phosphate depletion

B. Enhance tubular reabsorption
  1. Parathyroid hormone
  2. cAMP

Learn this table. Write it out at least 5 times with the book closed.

renin such as Kay-exalate (Resonium A) or calcium zeokarb 225 may cause hypomagnesaemia by binding magnesium. Diabetic ketosis may cause hypomagnesaemia due to excessive magnesium loss with the ketoacids as well with the glucose induced osmotic diuresis. Surgical drainage of fistula, the biliary tract, nasogastric suction or repeated drainage of ascites may cause hypomagnesaemia and magnesium depletion unless steps are taken to replace magnesium lost in suction or drainage. A simple rule is to consider that nasogastric suction or fistulae may cause a magnesium *loss of 1 mEq/l*. Remember this and read the last sentence again. Good.

Question A man with carcinoma of the prostate is found to have a serum calcium level of *3.5 mmol l^{-1}* or 14 mg/100 ml and a BUN of *3.3 mmol l^{-1}* or 20 mg/100 ml. What may his serum magnesium level be?

Answer 1. Low. Go on to **5.21**.
    2. Normal. Go on to **5.18**.
    3. High. Go on to **5.22**.

5.20   Your answer—30 mEq (*15 mmol*). This is a guess.

You should remember the rule in nasogastric aspirate there is 1 mEq of magnesium per litre. Now read **5.19** again.

5.21   Your answer—the serum magnesium is low.

Correct. Serum magnesium levels may be depressed in any patient with hypercalcaemia. Now let us suppose we have a patient with ileus who is having nasogastric aspiration for 2 weeks with intravenous replacement of fluids. The sodium, potassium and chloride content of the gastric aspirate is measured and replaced daily, but there is no atomic absorption flame photometer to measure serum magnesium levels. How much magnesium would you supply per day if you knew that his daily volume of gastric aspiration was 3500 ml?

Answer   1. 30 mEq (*15 mmol*) of magnesium a day. Go on to **5.20**.
2. 3.5 mEq (*1.75 mmol*) of magnesium a day. Go on to **5.23**.
3. 10 mEq (*5 mmol*) of magnesium a day. Go on to **5.25**.

5.22   Your answer—Serum magnesium level may be high.

You may have been correct if the hypercalcaemia had caused renal failure. However his BUN is normal, so you have made a poor guess. Hypercalcaemia of any cause, in man, may cause hypomagnesaemia. Read **5.19** again.

5.23   Your answer—3.5 mEq (*1.75 mmol*) of magnesium.

You are correct. Alcoholics develop hypomagnesaemia due to a combination of low dietary intake of magnesium and an increased urinary magnesium loss due to the effect of ethanol on the kidney. It causes an increased urinary excretion of magnesium. The cause of the very low plasma magnesium levels in severe hypoparathyroidism is probably the fall in tubular reabsorption of phosphate. It is postulated that the high plasma phosphate levels depress plasma magnesium levels as well as those of calcium. Therapy with vitamin D and magnesium is necessary before normal plasma levels of calcium and magnesium are obtained.

The clinical picture of magnesium deficiency, is mainly non-specific weakness, tremors, fibrillation of muscle and muscle fasciculation, tetany, and fits. There may be vomiting and paralytic ileus. It has been shown by MacIntyre that *pure* magnesium deficiency does not cause tetany, so that there are usually other factors such as hypocalcaemia, hypokalaemia or alkalosis. CNS changes are anxiety, delirium, and sometimes psychosis; choreoathetosis may develop. ECG changes are non-specific, and include nodal or sinus tachycardia, inverted T waves and ST depression. Fatal hypotension may develop in cases with profound magnesium deficiency— usually when plasma magnesium levels are 0.5 mg/l ($0.25 \, mmol \, l^{-1}$) or less.

Therapy of magnesium depletion and hypomagnesaemia. The therapy of hypomagnesaemia and magnesium deficiency is fairly straight forward. One gives an i.v. infusion of magnesium sulphate containing 50 mEq (*25 mmol*) of magnesium over 6 hours. **Remember that 1 g of magnesium sulphate** ($MgSO_4.7H_2O$) **contains 8 mEq** *(4 mmol)* **of magnesium** i.e. 4 ml of a 25 per cent solution of magnesium sulphate contains 8 mEq of magnesium, so that *25 ml of 25 per cent magnesium sulphate solution contains 50 mEq (25 mmol)*. This amount should be given in an intravenous drip over a period of 6 hours and not faster Plasma magnesium levels should be monitored carefully before the decision is made to continue this dosage or discontinue therapy because much of the inevitable loss of some of the administered magnesium (up to 80 per cent) through the kidneys and gut after injection.

Chronic hypomagnesaemia can be treated by oral magnesium oxide 250–500 mg/day (12.5 to 25 mEq/day or *6.25 to 12.5 mmol day^{-1}*) but may need to be limited by the diarrhoea which it induces.

Question How much magnesium in milliequivalents is there in 1 g of $MgSO_4. 7H_2O$?

Answer 1. 1 mEq. Go on to **5.24**.
          2. 8 mEq. Go on to **5.27**.
          3. 80 mEq. Go on to **5.26**.

5.24 Your answer—1 mEq/litre.
No. You are guessing. The answer is in **5.23**. You had better read it again.

5.25 Your answer—give 10 mEq (*5 mmol*) a day.
This is a sheer guess. Read **5.19** again which is full of facts. There is a simple rule of thumb for magnesium concentration in fistula fluids and nasogastric aspiration.

5.26   Your answer—80 mEq.
This is a guess. You have not recalled the salient fact that there each 1 g of $MgSO_4.7H_2O$ contains 8 mEq of magnesium. Read **5.23**

5.27   Your answer—8 mEq. This is *4 mmol in SI units.*
You are correct. Now answer the next question.

Question How quickly can you safely give 50 mEq (*25 mmol*) of magnesium intravenously in a patient with alcoholism and a serum magnesium level of 0.5 mg/100 ml (*0.2 mmol l^{-1}*)?

Answer   1. 24 hours. Go on to **5.28**.
            2. 2 hours. Go on to **5.30**.
            3. 6 hours. Go on to **5.32**.

5.28   Your answer—24 hours.
You are guessing. It is possible to give much higher rates of magnesium intravenously. Read **5.23** again then answer **5.27**.

5.29   Your answer—yes. Ethanol causes an increase in Mg loss.
You are correct. Having attempted to show that not too much is understood of magnesium metabolism in health, let us move on to disorders of magnesium metabolism. Magnesium deficiency is difficult to recognize apart from one of its manifestations—hypomagnesaemia. It has been already pointed out that hypomagnesaemia may be associated with a normal body magnesium content. Hypomagnesaemia is defined as a plasma magnesium level of less than *0.5 mmol l^{-1}* or 1.5 mg/100 ml (1.2 mEq/l). It may be caused by many things. These are listed in Table 5.29.
1. Inadequate intake of magnesium in the diet. In the ruminant this is a common condition and is known as grass tetany. It occurs in pastures in which magnesium is deficient, probably due to the ammonia in the young grass complexing magnesium so the magnesium is not absorbed in the gastro-intestinal tract. It is a major cause of death in ruminants in some areas. In humans, magnesium deficiency due to low magnesium intake occurs in protein calorie malnutrition, starvation, either economic or iatrogenic i.e. parenteral feeding for prolonged periods by doctors unskilled in their specialty. **Any patient receiving prolonged intravenous feeding (hyperalimentation) should have magnesium supplemented to his i.v. fluids.** Nasogastric suction is a potent cause of magnesium deficiency unless magnesium is replenished i.v. Severe

Table 5.29   Causes of magnesium deficiency (after Massry).

A. Decreased intake
  1. Protein–calorie malnutrition
  2. Prolonged parenteral nutrition

B. Decreased intestinal absorption
  1. Malabsorption syndromes
  2. Massive surgical resection of small intestine and by-pass operation
  3. Neonatal selective malabsorption of magnesium

C. Excessive losses of body fluids
  1. Prolonged nasogastric suction and parenteral fluids and laxative addiction
  2. Intestinal and biliary fistulas
  3. Severe diarrhoea as in ulcerative colitis and infantile gastro-enteritis
  4. Prolonged lactation

D. Excessive urinary losses
  1. Diuretic therapy—all natriuretic drugs
  2. Diuretic phase of acute renal failure
  3. Chronic alcoholism
  4. Primary aldosteronism
  5. Hypercalcaemic states: malignancy, hyperparathyroidism and vitamin D excess
  6. Renal tubular acidosis.
  7. Diabetes, especially during and following treatment of acidosis
  8. Hyperthyroidism
  9. Idiopathic renal magnesium wasting
  10. Chronic renal failure with renal magnesium wasting
  11. Gentamicin toxicity

E. Miscellaneous
  1. Idiopathic hypomagnesaemia
  2. Acute pancreatitis
  3. Porphyria with inappropriate secretion of antidiuretic hormone
  4. Multiple transfusions or exchange transfusions with citrated blood

---

Learn this table. Write it out at least 5 times with the book closed. Do not forget to do this.

diarrhoea of any cause will eventually cause magnesium deficiency. Surgical resection of the small bowel or short circuiting of the bowel for weight reduction also causes magnesium depletion.

Inability to absorb Mg from the GI tract occurs in malabsorption of any cause, steatorrhoeas being particularly noted for the formation of magnesium soaps by combination of magnesium with fatty acids. The magnesium in these soaps is not available for absorption by the bowel. Increased calcium intake such as can be obtained by taking 20 g of calcium lactate a day may impair magnesium absorption.

Urinary magnesium loss. In the normal person urinary magnesium excretion falls to about 1 mEq/day or 0.5 $mmol$ day^{-1} (12 mg) in the face of severe dietary magnesium restriction or magnesium deficiency.

An increased urinary loss of magnesium may cause magnesium depletion. These have been considered earlier but let us go over this important list once more.

1. Diuretics, including loop diuretics, osmotic diuresis and thiazides or any condition associated with sodium diuresis.
2. Hypercalcaemia and any condition associated with high urinary excretion of calcium.
3. Alcoholism (chronic).
4. Hyperaldosteronism—primary or secondary.
5. Hyperthyroidism.
6. Chronic renal failure.
7. Gentamicin toxicity.
8. Hyperparathyroidism.
9. Calcitonin therapy for hypercalcaemia or Paget's disease.
10. Renal tubular acidosis and diabetic ketosis.
11. Renal failure, acute or chronic with magnesium wasting.

Look at the list. Write it out. Memorize it. Now the renal compensation for magnesium deficiency is remarkably efficient. Urinary loss of magnesium falls to very low levels in magnesium deficiency of dietary origin. Intestinal secretion of magnesium continues during magnesium deficiency, so that dietary magnesium deficiency can be induced experimentally by a very low magnesium intake, despite excellent magnesium conservation by the kidney.

Question If a healthy person is given a diet containing no magnesium, what will his urinary magnesium excretion fall to?

Answer 1. 1 mEq/day (0.5 $mmol$ day^{-1}). Go on to **5.34**.
2. 10 mEq/day (5 $mmol$ day^{-1}). Go on to **5.36**.

5.30 Your answer—2 hours.
This will kill the patient and land you in jail. So please read **5.23** again, and read it very carefully.

5.31   Your answer——8–16 mEq (*4–8 mmol*).

You are correct. Good. Magnesium and calcium reabsorption are linked somewhat loosely. Thus sodium diuresis is paralleled by a magnesium diuresis and a calcium diuresis. PTH administration, cAMP administration, and magnesium deficiency all stimulate tubular reabsorption of magnesium in healthy animals. Ethanol administration causes an increased magnesium loss and sodium loss in the urine, but not a loss of calcium; this may explain the magnesium depletion seen in chronic alcoholics although inadequate diet is also a major factor. Magnesium excretion is increased in primary aldosteronism as well as in the first 90 minutes after administration of vasopressin during water diuresis. Administration of PTH causes a decreased excretion of magnesium, unless hypercalcaemia is present. PTH acts on the ascending limb of the loop of Henle, enhancing reabsorption of magnesium. Steroids cause a fall in magnesium excretion paralleling sodium retention. Chronic mineralocorticoid administration enhances magnesium excretion and giving the aldosterone inhibitor spironolactone prevents this. Growth hormone, calcitonin, thyroid hormone and vitamin D enhance magnesium diuresis. Generally whatever causes a sodium diuresis causes a magnesium diuresis. Thus the administration of loop thiazide or osmotic diuretics may cause eventual magnesium depletion due to magnesium loss paralleling sodium loss. Phosphate depletion enhances the loss of magnesium in the urine. Thus in alcoholics where phosphate depletion is common, there are several good reasons for the finding of magnesium depletion.

Question Does ethanol cause an increased urinary loss of magnesium?

Answer   1. Yes. Go on to **5.29**.
2. No. Go on to **5.35**.

5.32   Your answer——6 hours.

Good. You are correct. The renal handling of magnesium is in some ways similar to that of calcium, but less is known about it. Magnesium is filtered at the glomerulus, and because of protein binding 70 to 80 per cent of the plasma magnesium is non-protein bound and thus available for filtration through the glomerulus. Of this between 8 and 16 mEq per day appear in the urine i.e., about 5 to 10 per cent of the filtered magnesium load. It appears that 25 per cent is reabsorbed proximally and that 60 to 70 per cent is avidly reabsorbed in the ascending limb of the loop of Henle. This may be an active process or a passive process, merely a cation accompanying active chloride reabsorption at this site. There is little distal reabsorption of magnesium, although there is some evidence of magnesium secretion in the terminal portion of the collecting ducts in conditions of magnesium loading.

Question How much magnesium is found in the 24 hour urine collected from a healthy adult eating a normal diet?

Answer 1. 8–16 mEq(*4–8 mmol*). Go on to **5.31**.
　　　　 2. 50–100 mEq(*25–50 mmol*). Go on to **5.33**.

5.33　Your answer—50–100 mEq per day (*25–50 mmol*).
　　　That would be quite remarkable. It is unlikely that more magnesium would be excreted per day in health than is taken in a regular diet, I think you will agree therefore that you need to read **5.32** again carefully.

5.34　Your answer—1 mEq/day.
　　　You are correct. In acute pancreatitis, magnesium deficiency may be found, sometimes due to the i.v. infusion i.e. 'drip and suck' regime, possibly complicated by the formation of magnesium soaps similar to calcium soaps in the body fat due to liberated lipases. The magnesium in the soaps originates in the ECF and causes a fall in ECF magnesium levels akin to the similar changes in plasma calcium in this condition.
　　　Porphyria sometimes causes hypomagnesaemia, associated with SIADH — inappropriate secretion of antidiuretic hormone — which causes an increased loss of magnesium in the urine.

Question In a patient with acute porphyria, serum magnesium is 0.7 mg/100 ml (*0.3 mmol l^{-1}*) serum sodium 123 mEq/litre serum osmolality 245 mOsm/litre, urine osmolality 507 mOsm/litre, urine sodium 53 mEq/litre. What is the cause of his low serum magnesium level?

Answer 1. Diarrhoea. Go on to **5.37**.
　　　　 2. SIADH. Go on to **5.39**.

5.35　Your answer—No.
　　　Ethanol does not increase urinary loss of magnesium. You are not correct. Read **5.31** again and see what else you have day-dreamed through.

5.36　Your answer—10 mEq/day.
　　　No. This is the amount of Mg found in urine on a normal diet. You need to read **5.29** with greater concentration this time.

5.37 Your answer—diarrhoea.

No. In the question you are given enough data to make the diagnosis. Read **5.34** again, and stop day-dreaming. You can see that the patient has a serious hyponatraemia but a high urinary osmolality. Use your brain carefully.

5.38 Your answer—i.v. calcium gluconate.

You are correct. Now look at the following statements and think carefully before you choose the correct answer.

Statement 1 Magnesium is mainly found in the ECF.
Statement 2 Reticulocytes have lower Mg concentration than old cells.
Statement 3 Hypermagnesaemia is best treated quickly by i.v. calcium.

Your answer—1. All statements are true. Go on to **5.42**.
2. All statements are false. Go on to **5.51**.
3. Statement 1 is true, 2 and 3 false. Go on to **5.45**.
4. Statement 2 is true, 1 and 3 false. Go on to **5.46**.
5. Statement 3 is true, 1 and 2 false. Go on to **5.47**.
6. Statement 1 is false, the rest true. Go on to **5.48**.
7. Statement 2 is false, the rest true. Go on to **5.49**.
8. Statement 3 is false, the rest true. Go on to **5.50**.

5.39 Your answer—SIADH.

Good. You are correct. Addison's disease may be associated with hypermagnesaemia as well as hyperkalaemia and hypercalcaemia.

Magnesium excess is most frequently found in patients who have renal disease and thus have difficulty excreting the magnesium absorbed from the diet. Magnesium is absorbed normally in chronic renal failure, in contrast to calcium which is not absorbed due to its dependence on 1,25 dihydroxycholecalciferol which is not synthesized in the kidney in renal failure. As renal failure progresses there is an increasing bone content of magnesium and an increased red cell and muscle magnesium content. Normal red cell magnesium is 4.4 to 6.0 mEq/litre. Plasma magnesium levels rise with renal failure inconstantly, so that in any one patient there is no certainty that plasma magnesium levels will be abnormal; there is no direct connection between the plasma magnesium level and body stores of magnesium. Patients on regular haemodialysis often have raised plasma magnesium levels, especially if taking magnesium containing antacids or being treated with parenteral magnesium sulphate.

Hypermagnesaemia results in a reduced liberation of acetylcholine at the neuromuscular endplate, so blocking neuromuscular transmission. The symptoms of hypermagnesaemia are very variable. At around 6–8 mg/100 ml (5–7 mEq/l or *2.5 to 3.5 mmol l*$^{-1}$) there is cutaneous flushing due to vasodilatation and resultant hypotension. Drowsiness supervenes around a concentration of 10 mg/100 ml, (8 mEq/1 or *4 mmol l*$^{-1}$) and at this level there may be general weakness, loss of tendon jerks, and feeling of ill health. Muscular paralysis occurs at a level of around 12 mg/100 ml (10 mEq/1 or *5 mmol l*$^{-1}$) with coma at about 15–17 mg/100 ml (12 to 14 mEq/1 or *6–7 mmol l*$^{-1}$) and death due to respiratory depression. When errors in dialysate composition are made, plasma magnesium levels of 15 mg/100 ml (12 mEq/1 or *6 mmol l*$^{-1}$) have been seen with flushing of the face, fall in blood pressure, muscular weakness and dyspnoea. High levels may be found in the therapy of eclampsia with $MgSO_4$ which is obsolete and dangerous. Higher levels have been found after inhalation or swallowing of sea water (such as that in the Dead Sea) which is particularly rich in magnesium. This is usually fatal at levels of 16 to 17 mg/100 ml (13.3–14 mEq/l or *6–7 mmol l*$^{-1}$).

Question A man on regular haemodialysis is found to have predialysis serum magnesium levels of 8 mg/100 ml (6.7 mEq/l or *3.35 mmol l*$^{-1}$). What sort of phosphate binders is he likely to be taking?

Answer 1. $Al(OH)_3$. Go on to **5.41**.
         2. A mixture of $Al(OH)_3$ and MgO. Go on to **5.43**.

5.40 Your answer—i.v. saline.
    This will hardly help and by the time you a have finished putting up the i.v. infusion you will very possibly have a dead patient. Read **5.43** again.

5.41 Your answer—aluminium hydroxide.
    No. If you were correct, where is the patient getting such a high serum magnesium from? The answer is given in **5.39**. Read it. And if you cannot concentrate, close the book and do something else.

5.42 Your answer—all statements are true.
    Well if you think that, you have not learned anything from most of the chapter. Go back to **5.1**.

5.43 Your answer—a mixture of $Al(OH)_3$ and MgO.
    Correct. In the rat, magnesium deficiency is associated with *hyper-*

calcaemia and *hypo*magnesaemia. In man, however, *hypo*magnesaemia
is usually accompanied by *hypo*calcaemia. The hypercalcaemia in the
rat is most probably due to stimulation of parathyroid secretion. After
extirpation of the parathyroids, magnesium levels fall in the plasma, whereas after injection of PTH there is an increased urinary loss of magnesium
paralleling that of calcium. This is because the effect of hypercalcaemia
(causing hypercalciuria and decreased tubular reabsorption of Mg) over-
comes the *increase* in tubular reabsorption of magnesium caused by PTH.
Read this sentence again.

ECG changes include prolongation of the QT interval and prolonged
PR interval. AV block may be present.

Therapy of hypermagnesaemia. Calcium ion given i.v. in a dose of
10 ml of 10 per cent calcium gluconate over a period of 10 minutes
will antagonize the respiratory depression and cardiac arrhythmias of
hypermagnesaemia. Dialysis against a magnesium-free dialyzate should
then be applied in the case of hypermagnesaemia of renal failure. In non-
renal failure patients an i.v. saline/i.v. Lasix® diuresis (as used in
hypercalcaemia) is of benefit in ridding the body of magnesium. The dose
is 1 litre of saline and 40 mg of Lasix i.v. every 3–4 hours.

Question A patient has a serum magnesium of 12 mg/100 ml (10 mEq/l
or *5 mmol* l^{-1}) and has a PR interval of 0.24 seconds. What would you do
immediately on getting the results?

Answer 1. Give i.v. calcium gluconate. Go on to **5.38**.
       2. Give i.v. saline. Go on to **5.40**.
       3. Dialyse. Go on to **5.44**.

5.44 Your answer—dialyse.
While you are partially correct you may have a patient dying in the
time it takes to get the patient on dialysis. i.v. calcium may be life
saving. You should have picked this up in reading **5.43**. Go back and read
it carefully.

5.45 Your answer—statement 1 is true.
You are incorrect. Start again at the beginning of the chapter. There is
no point in deceiving yourself that you remember what you need to about
magnesium.

5.46 Your answer—statement 2 is true.
You are wrong. Start at **5.6** and work your way through the chapter.

5.47   Your answer—statement 3 is true.

You are correct. Now you can go on to the next chapter. You may want to look up some references.

Massey S. (1978) *Contributions to Nephrology* **14**, 64–73

Dirks J. (1978) In *Phosphate Homeostasis*. Massry, Ritz Rapado (ed) Plenum Press, New York.

Alfrey A. (1978) Magnesium. In *Renal Diseases and Electrolyte Metabolism*. R. Schrier (ed) Little Brown, Boston.

5.48   Your answer—statement 1 is false.

Yes, but so is statement 2. Start reading from **5.6** again. You must concentrate on learning.

5.49   Your answer—statement 2 is false.

That is correct, but you are wrong about statement 1. Read the first half of the chapter again and choose the correct answer in **5.38**.

5.50   Your answer—statement 3 is false.

That is wrong. You have got to read this chapter again from the beginning and concentrate on what you are learning this time.

5.51   Your answer—all statements are false.

No. Only the last is true. You ought to start reading at **5.33** again.

Chapter 6
Phosphorus

6.1 Phosphorus is found as either organic or inorganic compounds in the body. Organic compounds of phosphorus are of great importance in biological chemistry of all life forms—thus adenosine triphosphate is converted to ADP and a phosphate molecule with the liberation of energy: phosphate compounds of sugars such as diphosphogluconate, glucose 1 phosphate, glucose 6 phosphate, hexose monophosphate, pentosephosphates etc, all stress the importance of organic phosphorus compounds which occupy a key position in metabolism of nucleic acids and carbohydrates—the energy processes of the body are dependent on organic phosphorus compounds. However, the organic phosphorus compounds are only of interest in this course insofar as they are affected by or affect inorganic phosphorus metabolism. What is known of phosphate metabolism? The body stores of inorganic phosphorus are 600 g totally, of which 85 per cent are present in bone. Most of the remaining 15 per cent of phosphorus is inside the cells in compounds of carbohydrate, fat and protein intermediary metabolism. In the extracellular fluid there is about 600 mg (*19 mmol*). The normal plasma level of inorganic phosphorus (Pi) is 2.7 to 4.3 mg/100 ml (*0.87 to 1.4* mmol l^{-1}) in the adult, and in growing animals this figure is higher—thus in young children 5 to 6 mg/100 ml (*1.6 to 2.0 mmol l^{-1}* are commonplace. The higher the rate of growth of an animal the greater the plasma inorganic phosphorus concentration. This is because the plasma phosphate supplies the available substrate for synthesis of bone and organic phosphorus compounds.

Question What is the total amount of phosphorus in the body?

Answer 1. 600 mg. Go on to **6.3**.
2. 600 g. Go on to **6.5**.

6.2 Your answer—4:1.
Good. You are correct. Now let us have a look at bone.
In bone phosphate is present in hydroxyapatite $Ca_{10} (PO_4)_6 (OH)_2$. Part of the phosphate may be replaced by carbonate which is titrated off by excess hydrogen ion in renal failure, the carbonate of bone being a

major source of buffer in chronic metabolic acidosis of any cause. The following hormones influence inorganic phosphate metabolism:

1. Parathyroid hormone. This causes an increase in tubular rejection of phosphate i.e. decreased tubular reabsorption (TRP). TRP is normally measured as follows: after 3 days on a controlled standard phosphate diet a series of creatinine clearances and phosphate clearances (with 4 hourly urine collections) are obtained. The calculation is made as follows:

Measured   1. Plasma inorganic P = 4.0 mg/100 ml.
             2. Creatinine clearance = 120 ml/minute
             3. Urine phosphorus excretion = 0.4 mg/minute

Calculation   Filtered phosphorus $= \dfrac{120 \times 4}{100}$ mg/min = 4.8 mg/min

Now   Excreted load = 0.4 mg/min
       $\therefore$ Reabsorbed P = 4.8 − 0.4 mg/min = 4.4 mg/min
       $\therefore$ reabsorption of phosphorus $= \dfrac{\text{amt P reabsorbed}}{\text{amt P filtered}}$

= 4.4/4.8 = 0.916. You can try this calculation yourself in SI units. The answer for TRP should be the same.

The normal range is 0.85 to 0.95. This may also be expressed as a percentage i.e. 85 to 95 per cent. In man tubular reabsorption of phosphorus is decreased when there is increased parathyroid secretion. Thus it may fall to 0.40 or 0.30. In man TRP is not a particularly reliable measurement because of the influence of dietary phosphate intake, renal function and diurnal rhythms, on the test result.

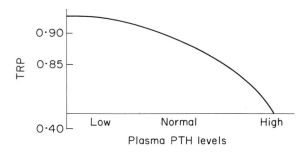

Fig. 6.2

Question A man has a TRP of 0.35. What is the diagnosis?

Answer 1. Hypoparathyroidism. Go on to **6.6**.
2. Hyperparathyroidism. Go on to **6.8**.
3. Normal parathyroid function. Go on to **6.10**.

6.3 Your answer—the amount of P in the body is 600 mg.
You are not correct. There are 600 mg of phosphorus in the ECF. The amount in the whole body is 1000 times greater. Read **6.1** again please.

6.4 Your answer—1:2. This is a guess.
Either you should sit still and learn sensibly, or close the book. If this early in the chapter you are unable to recall simple facts, you are distracted. Take appropriate steps to rectify this. Then go on to read **6.5** again.

6.5 Your answer—the amount of P in the body is 600 g.
Good, you are correct. The plasma phosphate is a mixture of HPO_4^{2-} and $H_2PO_4^-$ depending on the plasma pH. At a pH of 7.4 the ratio is approximately $HPO_4^{2-}/H_2PO_4^- = 4/1$. This variability is one of the reasons that it is more accurate to describe phosphate in terms of mg per 100 ml rather than in terms of milliequivalents per litre which require a precise knowledge of the proportions of HPO_4^{2-} and $H_2PO_4^-$ which are dependent on plasma and urinary pH, data on which are not necessarily available to the clinical biochemist who is expected to express his results in milliequivalents in some countries. In addition to phosphate there are plasma pyrophosphates in a concentration of 10^{-5} to 10^{-6} M which are important in inhibiting calcification; alkaline phosphatases may destroy pyrophosphates and so remove an inhibitor to calcification.

Question What is the ratio of HPO_2^{4-} to $H_2PO_4^-$ at pH 7.4?

Answer 1. 1:2. Go on to **6.4**.
2. 4:1. Go on to **6.2**.
3. 1:5. Go on to **6.7**.

6.6 Your answer—hypoparathyroidism.
No. This is not correct. Hypoparathyroidism gives a figure above the normal range, usually above 0.95 but not always so. Read **6.2** again.

6.7 Your answer—1:5.

Well that is a poor guess. If you are guessing you have not absorbed the material in **6.5** properly. Read it again.

6.8   Your answer—hyperparathyroidism.

You are correct. TmP, tubular maximum reabsorption of phosphate, can be measured in man but it requires intravenous phosphate loading and a simultaneous inulin clearance. TmP is depressed by glucose, bicarbonate and other anions. In man excess parathyroid hormone levels cause a fall in TmP. A rise in TmP is seen after parathyroidectomy. Also if parathyroid extract is given repeatedly there is a significant rise in TmP.

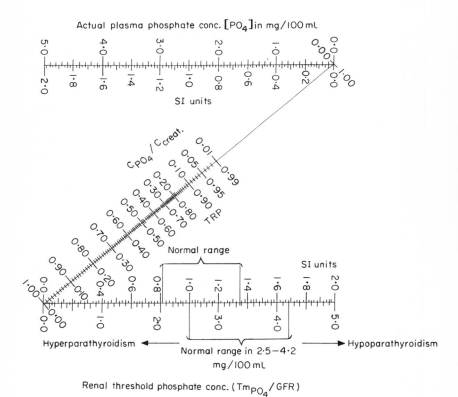

Fig. 6.8

Source: Modified from R. Walton and T.O.L. Bijvoet, *Lancet* **2**, 309, 1975.

Under conditions of eating a high phosphate diet there is a reduction of TmP.

To overcome the difficulty of measuring TmP directly Walton and Bijvoet introduced a nomogram which is shown here. Look at it. You need to know only plasma and urine phosphate and creatinine levels to obtain to ratio TmP/GFR. The normal range is 2.5–4.2 mg/100 ml. Above 4.2 mg/100 ml suggests hypoparathyroidism and below 2.5 mg/100 ml is suggestive of hyperparathyroidism. The ranges for SI units are also on the nomogram.

Phosphate clearance. This is calculated by the clearance formula

$C_P = UV/P$ where C_P = clearance of phosphate in ml/min.
$\qquad\qquad\qquad V$ = urine volume (ml/min).
$\qquad\qquad\qquad U$ = urine phosphate concentration (mg/100 ml).
$\qquad\qquad\qquad P$ = plasma phosphate concentration (mg/100 ml).

Mean normal $C_P = 10.8 \pm 2.7$ ml/min.
C_P usually is greater than 15 ml/min in primary hyperparathyroidism, but is affected by phosphate loading, diurnal rhythm and renal function. Now let us have a look at a question. A man with peptic ulcer and renal stones has the following blood and urine findings. Serum phosphorus 2.1 mg/100 ml $(0.7\,mmol\,l^{-1})$ urine vol 1440 ml/24 hours, urine phosphorus $13.6\,mmol\,l^{-1}$ or 42 mg/100 ml. His creatinine clearance is 120 ml/min. Calculate his phosphate clearance.

Answer 1. 200 ml/min. Go on to **6.11**.
$\qquad\qquad$ 2. 20 ml/min. Go on to **6.13**.
$\qquad\qquad$ 3. 20 mg/min. Go on to **6.15**.

6.9 How do you come to this paragraph? You have not followed instructions in answering the questions. Please do so or go to a conventional daydream-permitting book where you can fool yourself that you are learning.

6.10 Your answer—normal parathyroid function.
$\qquad$ You are not correct. The normal range of TRP is 0.85 to 0.95. The value in the question is 0.35. In your opinion is 0.35 equal to 0.85? Obviously not. What this tells you is that you are skimming. Forget daydreaming and speed reading. Learning facts takes time. Do not miss a word. Go over **6.2** carefully.

6.11 Your answer—200 ml per minute.

No, consider the clearance formula

$C = \dfrac{UV}{P}$ where $U = 42$ mg/100 ml

$P = 2.1$ mg/100 ml

$V = \text{ml/min} = \dfrac{1440}{1440} = 1\text{ml/min}$ $\therefore C = \dfrac{UV}{P} = \dfrac{42}{2.1}\text{ml/min.}$

Thus the answer is 20 ml/min. Go through **6.8** again.

6.12   Your answer—adenoma.

Most adenomas are autonomous, so you are wrong if you take the overall greatest likelihood. Read **6.13** more carefully this time.

6.13   Your answer—20 ml/min.

You are correct. Good. The patient probably has hyperparathyroidism, but he may have Fanconi syndrome or a variant showing abnormal tubular rejection of phosphate. This may not be the only tubular abnormality but the data are not given.

Phosphate Excretion index (P.E.I.). In this index devised by Nordin and Frazer, the level of serum P levels is taken into account, so bringing the filtered load of P into the calculation. Mass units i.e. mg/100 ml, *not* SI units, are used.

P.E.I. $= \underline{C_P} - 0.055 \times$ serum P $+ 0.7$

$\qquad\quad Ccr \qquad\qquad\qquad$ where $Ccr =$ creatinine clearance

normal values are between $= 0.09$ and $- 0.09$

P.E.I. is greater than $+ 0.09.$ in hyperparathyroidism and less than $- 0.09$ in hypoparathyroidism.

Index of Phosphorus Excretion (I.P.E.). This is a modification of P.E.I. This is a mass units calculation, *not* using S.I. units.

I.P.E. $= \dfrac{\text{P urine} \times \text{Serum creatinine}}{\text{urine creatinine}} - \dfrac{\text{P serum} - 2.5}{2}$

I.P.E. in normals is $- 0.5$ to $+0.5$

In hyperparathyroidism values of greater than $+ 0.5$ are found.

Calcium infusion test. Normal phosphate clearance is 10.8 ± 2.7 ml/min. On giving an intravenous infusion of calcium containing 15 mg of elemental calcium per kg body weight for a period of 3 hours, hypercalcaemia develops which causes the normal parathyroid hormone secretion to be suppressed. This results in a fall of phosphate clearance by 50 per cent. This is of course caused by an increase in tubular phosphate reabsorption when PTH levels fall. In patients with tumours causing primary hyperparathyroidism the fall in phosphate clearance is much less (i.e. 25 per cent) because the tumour is autonomous and is not sensitive to changes in plasma calcium; parathyroid hormone levels are unchanged in the face of increasing plasma calcium levels when an autonomous adenoma is present.

Question A calcium infusion test is given. The plasma immunoreactive PTH falls to immeasurably low levels and phosphate clearance falls from 20 ml to 7 ml. The patient is suspected of primary hyperparathyroidism. Is it more likely to be due to an adenoma or hyperplasia?

Answer   1. Adenoma. Go on to **6.12**.
2. Hyperplasia. Go on to **6.16**.
3. May be either. Go on to **6.17**.

6.14   Your answer—10 per cent.
No. If $20-40$ per cent of dietary phosphate appears in the faeces and the remainder is absorbed from the gut and appears in the urine, then it is fairly obvious what the answer is. Go back and read **6.16**.

6.15   Your answer—20 mg/min.
Almost correct. You have chosen the wrong units but done the calculation correctly. Clearance figures are given in ml per minute. Now go on to **6.13**.

6.16   Your answer—hyperplasia.
Correct. We have covered only a few of the phosphate tests in current use for the diagnosis of parathyroid disorders. Let us now look at phosphate metabolism in greater detail.
Dietary phosphorus intake is $900-1400$ mg/day. Of this $20-40$ per cent is excreted in the faeces, the remainder being absorbed from the gastro-intestinal tract and excreted in the urine.
Phosphate is absorbed from the stomach and small intestine. The more phosphate in the diet, the more is absorbed from the small

intestine and the more is then excreted in the urine. Phosphates in large doses attract water into the intestinal lumen and act as an osmotic cathartic.

Intestinal absorption from the small intestinal lumen can be by two routes.
1. Cellular mediated active transport.
2. Paracellular shunt pathway.

$1,25 \ (OH)_2 \ D_3$ stimulates active transport of phosphate and hence absorption from the intestinal lumen. Phosphorus absorption is sodium linked, 1 ion of Na^+ being absorbed with 1 ion of $H_2PO_4^-$.

In the plasma it has been claimed that about 10 or more per cent of phosphate is not filtered at the glomerulus because it is protein bound. Recent work in the rat does not substantiate this; it appears that none is bound. Of this filtered load of phosphorus only 5 to 10 per cent appears in the urine. The phosphate tubular maximum reabsorption capacity of the proximal tubule has already been discussed. It is set normally by levels of PTH in the plasma; the higher the plasma PTH levels the lower the TmPhosphate appears to be set. In a normal person if plasma levels of phosphate are lowered to 2 mg/100 ml ($0.7 \ mmol \ l^{-1}$) or less, say by phosphate depletion caused by the administration of phosphate binders such as aluminium hydroxide, then the urine is found to be phosphate free. Most, if not all, of the phosphate reabsorption takes place in the proximal tubule. Diseases of the proximal tubule, such as Fanconi syndrome, cause defective proximal tubular reabsorption of phosphate, causing an excessive loss of phosphate in the urine and a low plasma phosphate, as well as a loss of other substances which undergo proximal tubular absorption such as uric acid, glucose and amino acids: this results in a low plasma uric acid; renal glycosuria and amino-aciduria. In animals which are loaded with phosphate given in large amounts intravenously it has been claimed that overall tubular secretion occurs i.e. phosphate clearance is greater than inulin clearance, but this is still something which is disputed.

Question What percentage of dietary phosphate is found in the urine if the patient is taking a normal diet?

Answer 1. Up to 80 per cent. Go on to **6.19**.
         2. 10 per cent. Go on to **6.14**.
         3. None. Go on to **6.18**.

6.17 Your answer—may be either. You are correct but the most likely answer is hyperplasia i.e. which is still responsive to serum calcium levels. Read **6.13** again.

6.18 Your answer—none.

No. Phosphorus is always found in the urine of healthy people taking a normal diet. The reason for this is that up to 80 per cent of ingested P is absorbed and is excreted in the urine. Reread **6.16**.

6.19 Your answer—the urine has up to 80 per cent of dietary P.

Correct. Now answer the next question: If I gave a healthy man too much Al (OH)$_3$ as an antacid and his serum inorganic P level fell to 1.5 mg/100 ml, how much P would you expect him to excrete in his urine?

Answer 1. Very little. Go on to **6.20**.
   2. Normal amounts. Go on to **6.22**.

6.20 Your answer—very little phosphorus in the urine.

Good. You are quite correct. The level of inorganic phosphate in the plasma is the result of the interaction of parathyroid hormone, thyrocalcitonin, vitamin D metabolites, absorption from the gastro-intestinal tract, loss via kidney, and anabolism and catabolism of bone.

Extracellular fluid volume (ECF) expansion causes an increase in urinary phosphate excretion. *In vitro* in the perfused proximal tubule, glucose interferes with phosphate absorption, presumably by competition. Ouabain in the perfused renal tubule inhibits both glucose and phosphate absorption. The principal effect of parathyroid hormone on plasma phosphate is mediated via the kidney. PTH reduces tubular reabsorption of phosphate and causes increased loss of phosphate in the urine and consequently a fall in plasma phosphate levels. In its action on the kidney PTH liberates cAMP, the second messenger, which interferes with tubular phosphate reabsorption in the proximal tubule by the following: the cAMP activates protein kinase (at the brush border) which phosphorylates a protein transporting phosphate across the apical (luminal) cell membrane. cAMP is also activated by calcitonin and glucagon. Phosphate is absorbed from the tubular lumen *actively*, *against* an electrochemical gradient. When PTH acts on bone it liberates phosphate from the bone destroyed, and also hydroxyl ion. Thyrocalcitonin, on the other hand, causes bone anabolism with a fall in urine phosphate and a rise in plasma phosphate pari passu with a fall in serum calcium and a fall in urine calcium. Vitamin D acts on kidney, intestine and on bone via its metabolites 1.25 (OH)$_2$ Vit D$_3$ and 1:24:25 (OH)$_2$ Vit D$_3$. 1α OH D$_3$ has an antiphosphaturic effect caused by suppression of PTH secretion in the intact animal. P levels in plasma or tissues influence 1 α hydroxy-lase activity. 1 α hydroxylase converts 250H D_3 into 1.25 $(OH)_2D_3$. Phosphate depletion causes *decreased* tubular reabsorption of calcium: This may be due to partial secondary hypoparathyroidism.

Question ECF expansion causes what change in urinary phosphate excretion?

Answer 1. Increases urinary P excretion. Go on to **6.23**.
          2. Decreases urinary P excretion. Go on to **6.25**.

6.21 Your answer—PTH works directly on the renal tubule.
   No. It works via the liberation of cAMP, the second messenger. Read **6.20** again then answer **6.23** correctly.

6.22 Your answer—normal amounts.
   A reduction of available dietary phosphate by low P diet by a phosphate binding agent causes the formation of aluminium phosphate i.e. P not available for absorption—then the patient rapidly conserves P by absorption in renal tubules. Go back and re-read **6.16**.

6.23 Your answer—ECF expansion increases urinary P loss.
   Correct. Now answer the question.

Question Does PTH work directly on the renal tubule or through cAMP?

Answer 1. Directly. Go on to **6.21**.
          2. Through cAMP. Go on to **6.24**.

6.24 Your answer—PTH works indirectly through cAMP.
   Correct. Dietary phosphate intake is important as a contributing factor in phosphorus transport in the renal tubules. A low P diet causes a fall in urinary phosphorus; a high P diet causes a rise in urinary P excretion. This control occurs in parathyroidectomized animals, so it is not controlled by PTH. Nor is it controlled by ECF expansion, filtered load, pH, or vitamin D. This adaptation to dietary phosphorus takes 72 hours to be fully manifest, and the mechanism is unknown. Hyperphosphataemia is physiological in the growing young mammal. In childhood, levels of 5 to 6 mg/100 mg are normal. It is frequent in renal failure both acute and chronic, when plasma inorganic phosphate levels may rise to 20 mg/100 ml due to continuing absorption through the gastro-intestinal tract and from breakdown of cells without renal excretion of P being adequate.

In acromegaly there is an elevated plasma phosphate level. Hyperphosphataemia is asymptomatic unless the plasma calcium × plasma phosphate product is 70 or greater when both are expressed as mg per 100 ml. This is associated with metastatic calcification expressed acutely as 'red eyes' in renal failure or chronically as calcification at the limbus where the cornea joins the sclera between 2 o'clock and 4 o'clock. Look at Fig. 6.24I. The eyes are injected because of crystals of metastatic calcification—calcium phosphate in the epithelium causing conjunctivitis. In chronic metastatic calcification you need a lens and oblique light to demonstrate the sugar-icing like deposits in the conjuctiva. Metastatic calcification may occur elsewhere—most commonly in the blood vessels in the arteries most frequently, sometimes in the veins. Look at Fig. 6.24II. Renal metastatic calcification is frequent. This is known as nephrocalcinosis. Occasionally pulmonary and myocardial metastatic calcification is seen.

You will remember that action of parathyroid hormone on tubular phosphate reabsorption is mediated via cAMP. In pseudohypoparathyroidism, injection of PTH causes neither phosphaturia nor increased urinary cAMP in most cases. This is because of **end-organ unresponsiveness to parathyroid hormone.** In some patients cAMP is increased

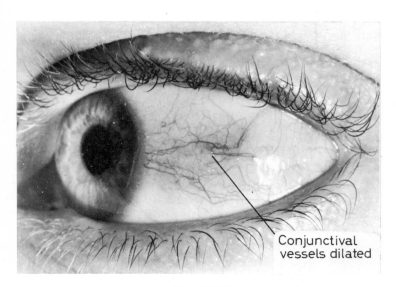

Conjunctival vessels dilated

Fig. 6.24I

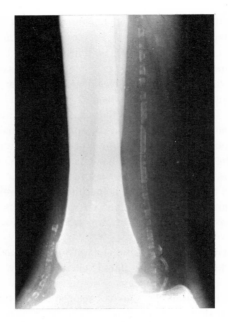

Fig. 6.24II

after PTH administration, suggesting a fault in response to cAMP in these patients.

Question In renal failure would you expect metastatic calcification if the serum Ca × P product was 55?

Answer 1. Yes. Go on to **6.26**.
2. No. Go on to **6.28**.

6.25 Your answer—ECF expansion decreases urinary P excretion. No. The answer is incorrect. Read **6.20** again.

6.26 Your answer—yes.
I would expect metastatic calcification. This is the wrong answer. Read **6.24** again, carefully this time and please concentrate. Otherwise shut the book and stop deluding yourself that you are learning. You are day-dreaming more than you are learning.

6.27   You cannot be following instructions if you are reading this. Go back and follow the programme.

6.28   Your answer—no.

I would not expect metastatic calcification. You are correct. The therapy of hyperphosphataemia is as follows:

1. Reduce phosphorus intake. This can be achieved by:

(a) Lowering phosphorus content of the diet itself—milk, eggs and meat are particularly rich in phosphorus. This can be achieved by a selected low protein diet i.e. the Giordano-Giovannetti diet.

(b) Giving a phosphate binder. This can be aluminium hydroxide, but there is some evidence that this is toxic in man. It gives rise to a type of resistant osteomalacia and to a dementia in patients on dialysis and is best avoided. Magnesium oxide has been suggested by Alfrey as a possible safe alternative but the absorption of magnesium in renal failure is unimpaired and consequently careful monitoring of serum magnesium levels is essential.

2. Use of more frequent dialysis is very advanced renal failure. Haemodialysis is carried out with a phosphate free dialysate. This results in a chemical gradient between blood and dialysis fluid so that plasma phosphate is lost into the dialysis fluid.

In childhood, hyperphosphataemia of 5 to 6 mg/100 ml (*1.6 to 2.0 mmol l*$^{-1}$) is normal, i.e. physiologic and should not be thought abnormal. It should *not* be treated. In acromegaly the therapy is that of the disease (operation, or deep X ray) rather than the hyperphosphataemia.

Question   If you find a boy of 7 has a serum phosphorus level of 6 mg per 100 ml (*2.0 mmol l*$^{-1}$) would you give him phosphate binders?

Answer   1. Yes. Go on to **6.30**.
          2. No. Go on to **6.32**.

6.29   Your answer—nutritional rickets.

You are correct. Now let us continue to examine hypophosphataemia in its milder form by discussing the causes of hypophosphataemia due to:

2. Urinary loss. (a) ECF expansion causes increased phosphaturia and thus phosphate depletion and hypophosphataemia.

(b) Diuretics—which increase sodium excretion also cause urinary phosphorus excretion to increase. Increase in urinary sodium excretion is usually associated with an increase in Ca, Mg and P excretion. This is the cause presumably of hypophosphataemia in prolonged Na HCO_3 therapy.

(c) Cortisone and hydrocortisone cause phosphate depletion.

(d) Recovery from hypothermia causes an increase in urinary phosphate excretion.

(e) Glucagon administration causes an increase in urinary phosphate excretion.

3. Shift of P into the cells. This is an interesting mechanism: hyperventilation causes a low serum phosphate by the following mechanism: lowering of Pco_2 causes an increase in cellular pH by lowering intracellular Pco_2. Thus stimulates intracellular glycolysis and phosphate enters the cells to form phosphorylated carbohydrate compounds. This causes a shift of P from plasma into the cells, and a mild fall in serum inorganic P. The conditions giving rise to a shift of P from plasma to cells are:

1. Salicylate poisoning.
2. Acute gout.
3. Gram negative bacteraemia.
4. Insulin administration.
5. Glucose administration.

Androgens cause a shift of P into the cells with incorporation of P inside the cells.

Question What is the cause of hypophosphataemia that is found in patients recovering from diabetic ketoacidosis who have received insulin.

Answer 1. Loss of P into the cells from ECF. Go on to **6.33**.
  2. Loss of P from cells into ECF. Go on to **6.35**.

6.30 Your answer—yes.

I would treat him with Phosphate Binders. You would be wrong and your answer tells me you have failed to absorb even one of the major facts in **6.28**. Go back and read it carefully. Do not day-dream. Do not try and speed read. You need to concentrate on every word.

6.31 Your answer—Fanconi Syndrome.

No. She has none of the hallmarks of this condition apart from a low serum phosphorus. The guess was a poor one. Read **6.32** more carefully.

6.32   Your answer—no.

I would not treat him. Correct. *Hypophosphataemia* is defined as a plasma inorganic P level of less than 2.7 mg/100 ml (*0.9 mmol l⁻¹*) in an adult. It has been subdivided by Massry into 2 groups: (a) Mild (Serum P = 1 to 2.5 mg/100 ml or *0.3 to 0.8 mmol l⁻¹*) (b) Severe— Serum P less than 1 mg/100 ml (< *0.3 mmol l⁻¹*)

Mild Hypophosphataemia has several main causes

1. Decreased intestinal absorption.
2. Increased urinary loss.
3. Shift of P into cells.
4. Combinations of the above.

Let us have a look at some causes of *mild hypophosphataemia*.
1. Increased urinary loss and decreased intestinal absorption of phosphate.

(a) Hyperparathyroidism. This has been mentioned earlier in Phosphate Tests and also in the chapter on calcium. Hyperparathyroidism may be primary or sometimes secondary. The diagnosis is discussed under phosphate tests, but if levels of serum iPTH levels (immunoreactive Parathyroid Hormone) are available, they are usually raised in both primary and secondary hyperparathyroidism. Calcium infusion does not usually depress serum iPTH levels in primary hyperparathyroidism due to tumour, but may depress hyperplastic glands. Hyperplastic glands are more frequent than adenoma in secondary hyperparathyroidism but this is not a 100 per cent reliable method of distinguishing—it leaves about 1 in 10 wrongly diagnosed.

(b) Osteomalacia due vitamin D deficiency (infantile and adult rickets): Hypophosphataemia is frequent in nutritional rickets, where it   is accompanied by hypocalcaemia and high plasma alkaline phosphatase. The urine is virtually calcium free. These abnormalities respond to administration of vitamin D. Hypophosphataemic vitamin D resistant rickets is due to a sex linked recessive gene. There is a primary defect in tubular phosphate reabsorption, with secondary hyperparathyroidism. Hypocalcaemia is not severe. Dwarfism is common, and unlike ordinary nutritional rickets, there is calcium in the urine in moderate amounts. Giving huge doses of vitamin D results in X ray healing of the rickets.

(c) Malabsorption   In this condition there is often the complication of vitamin D deficiency with low 25 OH D₃ levels.

(d) Fanconi Syndrome—amino phosphate diabetes: There are numerous causes—hereditary, heavy metal poisons, hyperglobulinaemias. All of them have multiple proximal tubular dysfunction—renal tubular glycosuria, low serum phosphate with a high phosphate clearance, low serum urate level with high urate clearance, amino-aciduria, and renal tubular acidosis.

Question A 16 year old Indian girl living in Glasgow, Scotland has pain in her back and limbs. Biochemical investigation gives the following results. Serum calcium is 7.4 mg/100 ml (*1.85 mmol l⁻¹*). Serum inorganic phosphorus is 2.5 mg/100 ml (*0.8 mmol l⁻¹*), she has an alkaline phosphatase which is increased and 25(OH)D₃ is 2 ng/ml, serum uric acid 6 mg/100 ml, urine sugar free. What is your diagnosis if X ray showed osteomalacia?

Answer 1. Nutritional rickets. Go on to **6.29**.
         2. Fanconi Syndrome. Go on to **6.31**.

6.33   Your answer—loss of P from ECF into cells.
     You are correct. Now let us move on to consider:

Severe hypophosphataemia.   What are the causes of severe hypophosphataemia, with serum Pi levels below 1 mg per 100 ml (*0.3 mmol l⁻¹*)? They are

1. Phosphate binding antacids.
2. Hyperalimentation without P replacement.
3. Recovery from burns.
4. Diabetic ketoacidosis.
5. Alcoholism C₂H₅OH causes loss of P in urine, there is little P in the diet of an alcoholic.
6. Severe respiratory alkalosis
7. Alcohol withdrawal, also associated with hyperventilation and thus causing a respiratory alkalosis and shift of P from plasma into cells. Also failure of replacing P lost in urine when on i.v. infusion.
8. Rehydration and refeeding with protein causes a massive need for P as anabolism proceeds. This is the same sort of mechanism as occurs in recovery from diabetic ketoacidosis, when severe P depletion develops due to entry of P into cells for anabolic purposes, so that ECF P levels fall dramatically, and severe P depletion ensues.

Learn this list. Write it down and make sure you know it. The presence of hypophosphataemia due to antacid abuse is caused by excessive amounts of aluminium hydroxide and magnesium oxide binding phosphate in the intestine so that a state of phosphate depletion occurs. Not only is dietary phosphate bound but also phosphate secreted into the intestine is also bound, so a very severe P depletion state develops. Therapy is cessation of phosphate binders. Give oral phosphates such as neutral sodium phosphate. Take care to keep the dose below that causing diarrhoea. Remember oral phosphates are osmotic cathartics. In severe cases it may be necessary to administer neutral phosphate mixtures of pH 7.4 intravenously, but this requires careful monitoring of plasma calcium levels to prevent serious hypocalcaemia developing.

Question When does the most hypophosphataemia appear in a chronic alcoholic?

Answer 1. Before admission to hospital. Go on to **6.36**.
2. In hospital, when he is being rehydrated and nourished intravenously. Go on to **6.37**.

6.34   Your answer—acute rhabdomyolysis.

Remember that acute rhabdomyolysis can be caused by injury, by coma usually due to drugs, by hypokalaemia, by hypophosphataemia and by McCardle's Syndrome.

In phosphate depletion, giving exogenous parathyroid hormone or expansion of the ECF volume gives a much blunted phosphate diuresis. *The metabolic acidosis of phosphate depletion is caused by a reduced tubular reabsorption of bicarbonate.* This results in a hyperchloraemic acidosis with a normal or reduced anion gap. What is the normal anion gap? It is 10 ± 2. Do you remember how to calculate it?

Anion gap = Serum Na minus the sum of serum chloride and bicarbonate. Ignore potassium. Its plasma value varies too much depending on plasma pH.

There is a reduced Tm glucose in phosphate depletion and because of the decreased phosphate excretion and low NH_4^+ excretion, there is a decreased titratable acidity. In hypophosphataemia there is an increase in the activity of 1α hydroxylase of 25 OH D_3. Lactic acidosis occurs in hypophosphataemia.

Now let us ask a question: Why is there a metabolic hyperchloraemic acidosis with a normal or low anion gap in phosphate depletion?

Answer 1. Decreased Tm HCO_3^-. Go on to **6.39**.
2. Lactic acidosis. Go on to **6.42**.

6.35 Your answer—loss of P from cells into ECF.

No. This is what happens in uncontrolled Diabetes Mellitus, but once it becomes controlled, insulin sends the P into the cells and so causes hypophosphataemia. Read **6.29** more carefully. Read every word. Bad choice of simple recall facts indicates lack of concentration. Find out why and correct it if you can.

6.36 Your answer—the worst hypophosphataemia appears before admission to hospital.

No. The answer is incorrect. However low the serum P level is on admission, we make it lower by rehydration, refeeding and so sending more P from ECF into cells for anabolism. You should have recalled this. Read **6.33** and see if you have missed anything else.

6.37 Your answer—the worst hypophosphataemia is manifest on treating him in hospital.

Good. You are correct. The effects of *mild* hypophosphataemia are not noticeable clinically. However, the *Effects of severe hypophosphataemia* are severe and may prove fatal. Let us divide them into clinical and laboratory features:

a. *Clinical*

1. *CNS*: irritability, dysarthria, hyperreflexia. Paraesthesiae, confusion, anisocoria, coma.

2. *Skeletal pains* and *pseudo-fractures on X ray* and sometimes fractures of pathological type i.e. with trauma which would not cause a fracture in a normal person.

3. *Muscular pain* and tenderness, weakness and paralysis, clinical signs of *rhabdomyolysis*.

4. *Cardiac failure* with decreased stroke volume and myocardial contractility and increased left ventricular end diastolic pressure.

b. *Laboratory Features*

1. *Blood*. Decreased red cell half life, with spherocytosis and rigidity of the red cell membrane, associated with haemolysis. The red cell ATP hexokinase and 2,3 DPG are reduced, and fructokinase and oxygen affinity are increased.

Leucocytes have abnormal function with reduced chemotaxis, phagocytosis and antibacterial activity. Thrombocytopenia with reduced platelet survival, and impaired clot retraction.

2. Hypoparathyroidism.

3. Liberation of phosphate and alkali from hydroxyapatite caused by breakdown of bone.

4. Elevated muscle CPK and aldolase.

5. Abnormal renal function and electrolytes. There is a reciprocal increase in serum calcium presumably liberated from bone. This is not due to PTH because there is a *secondary hypoparathyroidism due to inhibition of PTH secretion*. There is hypermagnesuria, as well as hypomagnesaemia. *Metabolic acidosis* is a constant accompaniment of phosphate depletion. Hypercalciuria is found in phosphate depletion. Phosphate virtually disappears from the urine.

Question   An alcoholic enters hospital and is treated for his acute or chronic alcoholism with i.v. fluids and oral feeding. One day it is noted that he has very high CPK (isoenzyme-muscle) and aldolase. Myoglobin is found in the plasma. He becomes very weak and his BUN rises to 150 mg/100 ml (*50 mmol l^{-1}*). Oliguria is noted. What has happened to cause his renal failure?

Answer 1. Sepsis. Go on to **6.40**.
            2. Acute rhabdomyolysis. Go on to **6.34**.
            3. Myocardial infarction. Go on to **6.38**.

6 38   Your answer—myocardial infarction.

No. Indeed I cannot say that he did not have an M I but there is no connection between that diagnosis and what you have been reading in **6.37**. Read **6.37** again and make the correct diagnosis.

6.39   Your answer—decrease Tm HCO$_3^-$.

You are correct. Now look at the following statements carefully before you pick the correct answer:

Statement 1. There are 600 g of phosphorus in the body.
Statement 2. PTH infusion causes an increase in tubular reabsorption of phosphorus.
Statement 3. Severe hypophosphataemia occurs during treatment of alcoholics.

Choose the correct answer:

1. All the statements are true. Go on to **6.41**.
2. All the statements are false. Go on to **6.43**.
3. Statement 1 is true, 2 and 3 false. Go on to **6.44**.
4. Statement 2 is true, 1 and 3 false. Go on to **6.45**.
5. Statement 3 is true, 1 and 2 false. Go on to **6.46**.
6. Statement 1 is false, 2 and 3 true. Go on to **6.47**.
7. Statement 2 is false, 1 and 3 true. Go on to **6.48**.
8. Statement 3 is false, 1 and 2 true. Go on to **6.49**.

6.40 Your answer—sepsis.
A very unusual answer and quite disconnected from the text. You really ought to read each paragraph more carefully. Reread **6.37**.

6.41 Your answer—all the statements are true.
You are incorrect about statement 2. Read up the renal physiology in section 1.2 before going on to the next chapter. Read **6.48**.

6.42 Your answer—lactic acidosis.
You are partly correct because lactic acidosis is found in phosphate depletion but it causes an increased anion gap, not a decreased or normal anion gap. Now answer the question in **6.34** correctly.

6.43 Your answer—all the statements are false.
No. Only 1 is false. Read through the chapter again.

6.44 Your answer—statement 1 is true.
Yes. But so is 3. Read the last third of the chapter again and go on to **6.48**.

6.45 Your answer—only statement 2 is true.
A bad guess. It is the only 1 wrong. Start the chapter again. If you want to know about phosphorus metabolism.

6.46 Your answer—statement 3 is true.
Yes, but so is statement 1. Read the first third of the chapter again then go on to **6.48**.

6.47 Your answer—statement 1 is false.
You are wrong. Start reading the chapter again.

6.48   Your answer—statement 2 is false, the remainder true.

You are correct. Now if you want to learn more about phosphate I would suggest you read the following books.

1. Massey S., Ritz E., Rapado A. (1978) Homeostases of Phosphate and other minerals. In *Advances in Experimental Medicine and Biology*. Vol. 103. Plenum Press, New York.
2. *Calcium Phosphate and Magnesium Metabolism* (1976) Edited by B. E. C. Nordin. Churchill Livingstone, London.
3. Lentz R., Brown D. M. and Kjellstrand C. M. (1978) Treatment of severe hypophosphataemia *Ann. Int. Med* **89**, 941–944.

6.49   Your answer—3 is false.

No. it is not correct. You need to read the chapter again but pay more attention to it.

Chapter 7
Acid–base balance

7.1 To begin with it is clear that the body pH has to be regulated between very narrow limits so that enzymes vital to metabolism can have their optimal conditions: small variations may lead to death or severe disability. It is therefore of paramount importance to understand the factors influencing acid base balance in health and disease so that one can understand what is happening in illness and how to treat it.

Let us start off at the beginning. The hydrogen atom contains a proton in its nucleus and an electron spinning around the nucleus. A hydrogen ion is formed by loss of the electron, and a proton remains, so that instead of the term hydrogen ion we may use the term proton. Thus acids are substances which ionize and liberate hydrogen ions or protons.

1. $HCl \rightarrow H^+ + Cl^-$.

They are called *proton* (i.e. hydrogen ion) *donors*. Bases are substances which combine with hydrogen ion i.e. *proton acceptors*.

2. $Na\,OH \rightarrow Na^+ + OH^-$
3. $OH^+ + H^+ \rightarrow H_2O$
4. $Na\,OH + HCl \rightarrow Na^+ + Cl^+ + H_2O$

The sum total of the reaction 4 has been the mopping up of the proton by the hydroxyl ion to form water. In fact hydrogen ion does not exist in body fluids as such, but is hydrated by combination with a molecule of water to yield H_3O^+ thus:

$$H_2O + H^+ \rightarrow H_3O^+.$$

In clinical medicine we refer to H_3O^+ as if it were a naked proton i.e. a hydrogen ion.

Hydrogen ions exist in very low concentrations in extracellular fluid and intracellular fluid. Indeed only in gastric acid do they approach 'normal' acid concentrations. In the plasma the free hydrogen ion concentration is of the order of 10^{-7} equivalents per litre i.e. 0.0001 mEq/l approximately. In arterial plasma the hydrogen ion concentration is 0.00004 mEq/l equivalent to what we will learn later is a pH of 7.4. In practice 0.00004 mEq/l is too small to use so that convenient units are nanoequivalents. Arterial plasma pH 7.4 is 40 nEq/l, with a range of 36–44 nEq/l i.e. pH of 7.44 to pH of 7.36. Memorize these figures. In the interstitial fluid i.e. the extravascular compartment of the ECF the hydrogen ion concentration varies from 3 to 25 nEq/l greater than in arterial blood. The range of hydrogen ion concentrations which are compatible with life is 20 to 120 nEq/l i.e. pH 7.7 to 6.9. The hydrogen ion concentration in intracellular fluids varies from tissue to tissue and from subcellular structure to structure. It is difficult to measure directly without tissue injury: indirect methods utilizing DMO have proved disappointing and controversial; suffice it to say that cells vary from 1000 nEq/l (pH 6.0) to 120 nEq/l (pH 6.9) depending on the cell and the method. However, some methods indicate intracellular hydrogen in concentration as high as 50 nEq/l (pH 7.3), but even this is of little meaning for the intracellular contents consist of discrete subcellular particles, each with its own anatomical and physiological characteristics, as well as the whirl of endoplasmic reticulum penetrating the cell.

Question What is the hydrogen ion concentration corresponding to a pH of 7.4?

Answer 1. 30 nEq/l. Go on to **7.3**.
2. 40 nEq/l. Go on to **7.5**.
3. 50 nEq/l. Go on to **7.7**.

7.2   Your answer—pH.
No. You are guessing. And a poor guess. Go back to **7.5** and read it carefully and without distraction.

7.3   Your answer—30 mEq/l.
You are not correct. You have not concentrated while reading **7.1**. Read it again more carefully. 30 mEq/l corresponds to a more alkaline pH than 7.4.

7.4   Your answer—P_{CO_2}.
No. You have made a poor guess. This is early in the chapter and you should be learning most efficiently in the first 15 minutes. Please start again at **7.5** but concentrate.

7.5   Your answer—40 nEq/l.
You are correct. Good. Thus whatever method we use in measuring

intracellular hydrogen ion concentration is doomed to be fairly meaning-less when considered in the light of the ultrastructure of the cell. This applies to all cells, although the subcellular particles differ in the various cells according to their respective functions. So remember that intra-cellular fluid is not a homogeneous entity but is made of multiple com-partments each with its own characteristics anatomically and bio-chemically.

There are 3 major methods of physiological control of the hydrogen ion concentration in the body fluids, namely,

1. Body buffers.
2. Respiratory regulation of CO_2 concentration in the body.
3. Renal mechanisms.

Before we consider the buffer systems in the body let us revise what the term buffer means: a buffer is a system of mopping up hydrogen ions or hydroxyl ions which are added to the system so as to minimize any change in hydrogen ion concentration. In the body ECF, hydrogen ion concentration may also be maintained by another type of buffering i.e. where the hydro-gen ion is transferred *out* of the ECF so that the ECF hydrogen ion content remains constant at the *expense* of intracellular mechanisms for dealing with hydrogen ion which has penetrated into the cells from the ECF. The time taken for this transfer of H^+ out of the ECF and into the cells is at least 2 hours, so that when treating high hydrogen ion concentrations in the ECF with intravenous bicarbonate one should expect that *complete* hydrogen ion equilibrium will take 2 hours at least, although for practical purposes 2 hours is adequate, as in any case hydrogen ion is being con-tinually generated metabolically in the cells at the same time.

What is the buffering system in man? The first and most important buffer is the blood. The blood buffering power is composed of several separate buffers:

1. bicarbonate in plasma and red cells,
2. haemoglobin,
3. plasma proteins,
4. phosphate in plasma and red cells.

Of the buffers in blood the bicarbonate and haemoglobin are of major importance. The bicarbonate buffer system links in to the respiratory control of hydrogen ion. Let us look at the bicarbonate buffering system.

$$H_2O + CO_2 \overset{CA}{\rightleftharpoons} H_2CO_3 \rightleftharpoons H^+ + HCO_3^-$$

The letters CA indicate the activity of the enzyme carbonic anhydrase which is responsible for catalyzing this reaction i.e. hydration of CO_2 to carbonic acid. In the presence of carbonic anhydrase in blood the reaction proceeds so fast that the limiting factor is the diffusion of CO_2. The concentration of H_2CO_3 is most conveniently measured by measuring the P_{CO_2} with an electrode and multiplying the P_{CO_2} by 0.03, the results being in mmol/l.

Thus H_2CO_3 is expressed in terms of dissolved CO_2 as mmol/l.

For example:

$P_{CO_2} = 40$ mmHg

Therefore dissolve $CO_2 = (H_2CO_3) = 40 \times 0.03$ mmol/l

$$= 1.2 \text{ mmol/l}$$

There are normally 26–32 mmol of bicarbonate in each litre of plasma.

$$(H^+) . (HCO_3^-) = K (H_2CO_3)$$

$$(H^+) = K \frac{(H_2CO_3)}{(HCO_3^-)} .$$

If $-\log H$ is called pH

$$\text{then pH} = pK + \log \frac{(HCO_3^-)}{(H_2CO_3)} .$$

Now this is known as the Henderson–Hasselbalch equation—not Hasselblach or Hasselbach, but *Hasselbalch*. Do not forget it. It is the least tribute to remember the name of one of the men who thought up the idea.

Now pKa for carbonic acid is 6.1.

In a normal man the arterial pH can be determined from the bicarbonate

1. $\text{pH} = 6.1 + \log \dfrac{HCO_3^-}{H_2CO_3}$

2. $\text{pH} = 6.1 + \log \dfrac{24}{1.2}$

3. $\text{pH} = 6.1 + \log 20$

4. $\text{pH} = 6.1 + 1.3$

5. $\text{pH} = 7.4$

Now when $\dfrac{\text{Base}}{\text{Acid}} = 1$,

then $\text{pH} = pK$.

A buffer is most active at buffering (i.e. its effect at minimizing hydrogen ion changes is greatest) within $\frac{1}{2}$ a pH unit on either side of its pK value. Look at the pKa for various materials found in blood:

Substance	pKa
Carbonic acid	6.1
Phosphoric acid (pKa$_2$)	6.8
Creatinine	4.8

Thus carbonic and phosphoric acids have useful pKa values from the point of view of buffering blood which has a pH of from 6.9 to 7.7 at its widest extremes beyond which life cannot be supported. With regard to buffering urine, creatine can also be seen to be within the physiological range of urine pH (from pH 4.6 to pH 8.4).

Question What indicates the pH at which there is maximum buffering capacity of a buffer?

Answer 1. pH Go on to **7.2**.
  2. Pco_2 Go on to **7.4**.
  3. pK Go on to **7.8**.

7.6 You should not be reading this if you are following the programmed instructions.

7.7 Your answer—50 mEq/l.
  You are not correct. 50 mEq/l is more acid than pH 7.4. This is a failure of immediate recall of a simple fact and indicates that your learning is faulty. Start **7.1** again.

7.8 Your answer—pK.
  You are correct. Now answer the question. What is the pKa of carbonic acid. Do not look back to **7.5**. Choose the answer.

Answer 1. 6.8. Go on to **7.9**.
  2. 6.1. Go on to **7.11**.
  3. 4.8. Go on to **7.13**.

7.9   Your answer—6.8.

No. Your memory is faulty. That means either you are not concentrating or that you are tired. I assume that if you are wise enough to buy and read this book then you are not demented. Read **7.5** again carefully, and answer question **7.8** again.

7.10   Your answer—reduced haemoglobin.

You are correct. Now let us look at *respiratory control of acid–base balance*.

The unique property of bicarbonate as a blood buffer is its ability to control body CO_2 content by means of lung regulation. P_{CO_2} can be readily lowered by increasing the rate and/or depth of breathing: P_{CO_2} can be elevated by decreasing the rate and/or the depth of breathing in normal man. Now the concentration of CO_2 in the blood depends on the loss of CO_2 from the lungs. In normal helath there is a direct correlation between CO_2 production in the tissues and loss of CO_2 via the lungs. In man there are about 20 equivalents of CO_2 produced each day i.e. 20,000 mEq that are excreted via the lungs. This is an immense quantity which can be varied according to the needs of the body. If excess hydrogen ion is added to the body fluids then it reacts with bicarbonate to produce CO_2 which can be excreted through the lungs and so the excess H^+ has been buffered.

$$H^+ + HCO_3^- \rightleftharpoons H_2CO_3 \rightleftharpoons H_2O + CO_2.$$

Similarly if OH^- is administered, then the reaction goes in the reverse way, CO_2 being used to produce carbonic acid which liberates hydrogen ion: the hydrogen ion then combines with hydroxyl ion so preventing any change in the hydrogen ion concentration of the ECF.

$$CO_2 + H_2O \rightarrow H_2CO_3 \rightarrow H^+ + HCO_3^-$$
$$H^+ + OH^- \rightarrow H_2O.$$

The excess bicarbonate is dealt with by renal mechanisms. For the above reaction CO_2 is available from the 20 equivalents produced metabolically each day, but if OH^- has been administered to the subject only by a reduction in ventilatory rate and/or depth may it be possible to maintain the pH normal by using the CO_2 which is continually produced. This is *respiratory compensation of an alkalosis*.

Question How much CO_2 is produced a day?

Answer 1. 20 mEq. Go on to **7.14**.
2. 20 equivalents. Go on to **7.16**.
3. 20,000 mEq. Go on to **7.18**.

7.11   Your answer—pK 6.1.
Good. You are correct.

Note at this stage that pH is written with a small p to signify negative logarithm, whereas $P\text{co}_2$ is written with a capital P to denote partial pressure—do not confuse the two please. Even reputable scientific journals mix them up, but it is an error akin to calling a man 'Mrs.'. Don't do it.

So what? How does bicarbonate act as a buffer system? Well, if we add hydrogen ion to the blood it combines with bicarbonate in the plasma, forming carbonic acid which is rapidly transformed

$$HCO_3^- + H^+ \rightleftharpoons H_2CO_3 \rightleftharpoons H_2O + CO_2$$

under the influence of carbonic anhydrase in the red cells to water and carbon dioxide. The carbon dioxide is blown off by the lungs by means of a particularly sensitive method of control of plasma $P\text{co}_2$ in normal health. Thus if we add 14 mEq of acid to the blood of a dog, with the bicarbonate buffer system the pH, which would have fallen to 6.06 on theoretical grounds, is found to be 7.10 solely due to increased loss of CO_2 by the lungs. This is *respiratory compensation of a metabolic acidosis*. It works the opposite way in metabolic alkalosis, CO_2 being retained and the rise in blood pH minimized.

It is thus apparent that the carbonic acid/bicarbonate system of buffering in the blood is intimately connected with the respiratory control of hydrogen ion content of the ECF.

A convenient way to obtain the Hydrogen ion *Concentration* is by use of the equation of Kass:

$$(H^+) = 24 \times \frac{P\text{co}_2}{HCO_3^-} \qquad \text{where } P\text{co}_2 \text{ is in mmHg}$$
$$HCO_3^- \text{ is in mmol/l}$$
$$H^+ \text{ is in nEq/l.}$$

or alternatively we can obtain $P\text{co}_2$ from bicarbonate by the following $P\text{co}_2 = 1.5 \ (HCO_3^-) + 8$.

The haemoglobin buffer is quantitatively as important as the carbonic acid/bicarbonate buffer system. Thus the buffering power of *1 litre* of blood is as follows:

Reduced haemoglobin—27.5 mEq of hydrogen ion.
Plasma proteins—4.2 mEq of hydrogen ion.

Reduced haemoglobin is a stronger base than oxyhaemoglobin i.e. it has a stronger capacity to combine with hydrogen ion. Haemoglobin therefore mops up the hydrogen ion more readily in the tissues pari passu with giving up its oxygen, so that it is a particularly effective buffer where it is most needed, i.e. where H^+ is being liberated. It buffers the H_2CO_3 being formed in the tissues particularly effectively

$$H^+ + Hb^- \rightarrow HHb.$$

The action of phosphate as a blood buffer is particularly interesting:

Now phosphate can exist in 3 forms: PO_4^3 HPO_4^2, $H_2PO_4^-$.

At the pH of blood only the sytem $HPO_4^{2-}/H_2PO_4^-$ has a pKa of 6.8 which is close enough to that of blood to be of importance as a buffer i.e. half a pH unit on either side of the pKa. Creatinine you will recall has a pKa too low to be of significance as a buffer in the blood. One should bear in mind that the blood buffers are not solely plasma but that haemoglobin, bicarbonate and phosphate, are found in the red cells and act as important blood buffers from that site.

Question Which buffers more hydrogen ion per litre of blood?

Answer 1. Reduced haemoglobulin. Go on to **7.10**.
2. The plasma proteins. Go on to **7.12**.

7.12 Your answer—The plasma proteins.
No. They only can buffer about 4 mEq of H^+ per litre. You need to read **7.11** again.

7.13 Your answer—4.8.
No. You are guessing. You cannot remember some very important facts in **7.5**. Go back and read them very carefully. If you have distractions, turn them off or stop reading. You cannot learn about electrolytes any other way than by absorbing the salient facts from this book. Then you will understand what is going on clinically much better. So please try to learn **7.5** and then choose the correct answer in **7.8**.

7.14 Your answer—20 mEq.
You are wrong. The correct answer is 1000 times greater. Read **7.10** again.

7.15 Your answer—4000 mEq a day.
Correct. Good.

Now what is titratable acid in the urine? If the urine is titrated up from its acid pH, for example, 4.9, to the pH of plasma 7.4, using normal sodium hydroxide we can derive from the quantity of sodium hydroxide needed, the amount of buffering capacity of the urine. This is known as the titratable acidity of the urine and consists of two main components:

(a) $H_2PO_4^-/HPO_4^{2-}$ —the urinary phosphate buffering system where HPO_4^{2-} can remove hydrogen ion as follows:

$$HPO_4^{2-} + H^+ \rightleftharpoons H_2PO_4^-.$$

This has a pKa of 6.8 and is thus active over the range 7.3 to 6.3.

(b) Creatinine. This has a pKa of 4.8 and is thus of considerable importance in the buffering power of urine near the lower end of the pH range.

Both phosphate and creatinine are limited in their buffering power by their quantity in the urine—this is a function of glomerular filtration and in the case of phosphate, tubular reabsorption and possibly, under certain circumstances tubular secretion as well. It is clear that titratable acidity cannot be increased by the appearance of more phosphate in the urine than can be filtered at the glomerulus, but that the amount of hydrogen ion being picked up by the phosphate depends on the degree of urinary acidification.

Urinary ammonium. When titratable acidity is measured the hydrogen ion which combines with ammonia (to form ammonium ion) is not liberated

$$NH_3 + H^+ \rightarrow NH_4^+$$

and thus does not neutralize the sodium hydroxide and is therefore not measured as titratable acidity. Nevertheless urinary ammonia is an important mechanism of excretion of hydrogen ion. Ammonia itself combines with hydrogen ion to yield ammonium ion:

$$NH_3 + H^+ \rightarrow NH_4^+.$$

The ammonia is a gas similar to this sense to CO_2 with a measurable partial pressure (P_{NH_3}). It can diffuse freely through the lipid tubular cell membrance. When ammonia gas gets into the tubular fluid it combines with hydrogen ion secreted into the lumen from tubular cells and forms ammonium.

The formation of ammonium ion results in a lowered P_{NH_3} in the tubular fluid so that more NH_3 leaks across the lumen into the fluid and more is neutralized by the hydrogen ion being secreted. The ammonium

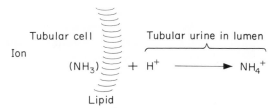

Fig. 7.15

ion is charged positively and is unable to penetrate the renal tubular cell wall, whereas the non-polar NH_3 gas is able to penetrate the tubular cells easily. This is known as *non-ionic diffusion* and is the mechanism responsible for the gradient of ammonia from tubular cell into tubular lumen.

Question Is NH_4^+ lipid soluble?

Answer 1. Yes. Go on to **7.19**.
2. No. Go on to **7.20**.

7.16 Your answer—20 equivalents.

You are correct. Let us go on to *Renal Control of Acid–Base Balance*.

The kidneys are the major organs of excretion of inorganic and organic ions either produced by catabolic processes in the body or ingested. In the normal human kidney 5000 mEq of bicarbonate is filtered each day. If the urine pH is less than 6.2 no bicarbonate at all is found in the urine, so 5000 mEq must have been reabsorbed. If the pH of the urine is above 6.2, increasing amounts of bicarbonate are excreted. 85 per cent of bicarbonate is reabsorbed in the proximal tubule. HCO_3^- reabsorption is clearly (3) dependent on (1) the volume of the ECF, (2) potassium, (3) P_{CO_2}. These will be discussed later. The distal tubule has a clearly defined $TmHCO_3$ which is readily overcome if more bicarbonate fails to be reabsorbed proximally.

The body produces about 50–70 mEq of hydrogen ion each day from catabolism of protein: (such as phosphoproteins and methionine) which are metabolically equivalent to phosphoric acid and sulphuric acid respectively. The hydrogen ion which is so formed is excreted by the healthy kidney by the following means:

1. As titratable acid. The glomerular filtrate commences at the hydrogen ion concentration of plasma but when it is passed as urine its pH may vary from 4.6 to 8.3. At a pH of 4.6 the ratio of hydrogen ion in urine to that in the blood is 800 to 1. The hydrogen ion has been added in the proximal or distal tubule. First of all in the proximal tubule hydrogen ion is added in the reabsorption of bicarbonate thus:

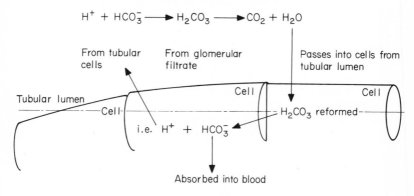

Fig. 7.16

Look at the diagram. You will see that as a net result of hydrogen ion secretion into proximal tubule filtered bicarbonate is absorbed into the proximal tubular cell from the lumen and thence into the blood. Virtually all of the bicarbonate in the proximal tubule may be absorbed this way. Let us see how much this is. If the bicarbonate level in the plasma is 25 mmol l^{-1} i.e. 2.5 mmol/100 ml and the GFR is 120 ml/min then each minute 2.5×1.2 mmol of bicarbonate are absorbed. i.e. per day $2.5 \times 1.2 \times 1440$ mmol are absorbed i.e. 4320 mmol per day. Now for each mmol of bicarbonate reabsorbed 1 mEq of H^+ has to be secreted, so that in bicarbonate reabsorption alone 4320 mEq of hydrogen ions are secreted into the renal tubules each day 80—90 per cent of this is secreted obligatorily into the proximal tubule, the remainder being secreted into the distal tubule according to the variable requirements of the body. If it is necessary to secrete an acid urine, and a urine of pH less than 6.2 is elaborated, the urine will be free of bicarbonate because all the bicarbonate remaining in the distal fluid will have combined with secreted hydrogen ion and thus have been reabsorbed. Only with urine of pH greater than 6.2 is bicarbonate found in the urine. This can be readily demonstrated in alkaline urine when the salicylsulphuric acid test is used for detection of protein. When the acid is first added to the urine, bubbles of CO_2 come off—the urine effervesces—until the bicarbonate has all been titrated by the acid.

7.16 **Question**   How much bicarbonate is reabsorbed per day in the kidney?

Answer 1. Over 4000 mEq. Go on to **7.15**.
2. Over 400 mEq. Go on to **7.17**.

7.17   Your answer—400 mEq a day.
No. You are out by a factor of 10. Read **7.16** again.

7.18   Your answer—20,000 mEq.
You are correct. Go on to **7.16**.

7.19   Your answer—NH_4^+ is lipid soluble.
No. Were it lipid soluble, much of what you have read in **7.15** would be nonsense. No. You have not paid attention to your reading. Kindly do so. Reread **7.15**.

7.20   Your answer—NH_4^+ is not lipid soluble.
Good. You are correct. The source of the ammonia secreted from the tubular cell is the tubular cell itself, for the concentration of ammonia in the renal vein is greater than that in the renal artery. Therefore it must be produced in the kidney. Ammonia is produced mainly from the amide nitrogen in glutamine in the kidney by the following:

1. Splitting of glutamine under the influence of glutaminase I
glutamine $\xrightarrow{\text{glutaminase I}}$ glutamate $+ NH_3$
2. Glutamate oxidation: glutamate $+ O_2 \rightarrow$ ketoglutarate $+ NH_4^+$
3. *Deamination* of glutamine under the influence of glutaminase II
glutamine $+$ ketoacid glutaminase $\xrightarrow{\text{glutaminase II}}$ ketoglutaramate
4. Ketoglutaramate $\rightarrow$ ketoglutarate $+ NH_3$.

The amount of ammonium produced in the kidney and excreted in the urine depends on the following factors:

1. Glutamine available—i.e. substrate available.
In renal failure less functioning kidney tissue is present and so less substrate is available.
2. Sodium is exchanged in the distal tubule for hydrogen ion. The more sodium reabsorbed the more hydrogen ion is liberated into the tubular lumen and is thus capable of combining with NH_3 in the lumen to yield NH_4^+.

In man a fall in urine pH associated with acid ingestion is associated with increased ammonium in the urine; this is also found in respiratory acidosis. Alkaline urine resulting from potassium loading, sodium bicarbonate administration or diamox (acetazolamide) administration decreases NH_4^+ excretion. There is a good correlation between NH_4^+ excretion and urine pH; this is particularly marked in potassium depletion. In chronic acidosis glutaminase production is induced and more NH_4^+ is found in the urine than at the corresponding pH in normal non-acidotic animals.

The ammonia excretion per ml of GFR is relatively normal in advanced renal failure, but because GFR is so reduced (20) then overall ammonia excretion per kidney is much reduced similarly overall. Phosphate excretion is reduced because of the reduction in phosphate filtered at the glomeruli caused by the loss of functioning glomeruli.

The quantity of ammonia excreted per day is usually $30-40$ mEq/24 hours. This is particularly important in infancy where titratable acid is low and most of the hydrogen ion is excreted as ammonium. In the adult about half is excreted as ammonium and half as phosphate.

Total hydrogen ion excretion is given by the following formula:

$$H^+ = \text{(Titratable acidity)} + (NH_4^+) - (HCO_3^-)$$

where H^+ titratable acid, NH_4^+, HCO_3^- are expressed as mEq/day.

Titratable acidity, you will remember, is largely due to the conversion of HPO_4^{2-} to $H_2PO_4^-$ i.e. the trapping of hydrogen ion on phosphate. Ammonium is also obviously a mechanism of trapping H^+ as NH_4^+. Why is the 'minus bicarbonate' included in the total H^+ formula? It is included for technical reasons because if there is a pH of urine of less than 6.2 there is no bicarbonate and titration with NaOH directly to pH 7.4 gives us the titratable acidity. If there is a pH of 6.2 or more and bicarbonate is found in the urine, then this has to be neutralized first by titration with acid and the result obtained is titratable acid minus bicarbonate. Bicarbonate is metabolically equivalent to hydroxyl ion (OH^-) and so can be considered to be negative hydrogen ion, so that when calculating total urinary excretion of hydrogen ion, one is obliged to include HCO_3^- as negative H^+.

Question How much NH_4^+ is found in the urine per 24 hours in a normal adult.

Answer 1. 30—40 mEq. Go on to **7.22**.
2. 1—3 mEq. Go on to **7.24**.
3. None if the urine has a pH which is high. Go on to **7.82**.

7.21 Your answer—there is a decrease in H⁺ in the cells.

No. If K is lost from the cells some other cations enter, one of which is hydrogen ion. Read **7.22** again.

7.22 Your answer—30—40 mEq.

Good. You are correct. In normal health the lowest urinary pH found is about 4.6. However, a lower pH, down to 4.1, has been recorded if a non-reabsorbable anion is given intravenously, such as ferrocyanide or sulphate, in state of induced sodium depletion. The mechanism of this is interesting; sodium ferrocyanide or sulphate enters the distal tubule and the sodium ion is reabsorbed: H^+ and K^+ are secreted in exchange to accompany the non-reabsorbable anion. Thus the urine is of low pH and also the hydrogen ion excreted combines with HPO_4^{2-} to yield $H_2PO_4^-$ with a resultant increase in titratable acidity. If reabsorbable anion only is present then it is absorbed with the sodium without the excretion of large amounts of hydrogen ion and potassium ion because there is no massive amount of unreabsorbable anion present in the tubular lumen which must obligate the presence of cation to maintain electrical neutrality. If there is a deficiency of chloride in the distal tubule due to hypochloraemia e.g. caused by vomiting or by continued use of diuretics, then chloride is not available for reabsorption with sodium and if the anions which are occupying the space of the absent chloride—phosphate, bicarbonate or organic acids depending on the circumstances, are reabsorbed

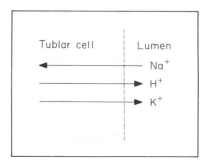

Fig. 7.22

then there is an increased loss of potassium ion and hydrogen ion in the urine. This results in a hypokalaemic alkalosis in diuretic induced chloride depletion; correction of the hypokalaemic alkalosis is contingent on the administration of chloride as well as potassium. This is because the chloride ion reaches the distal tubule in sufficient quantity to accompany sodium ion back into the tubular cell; this conserves potassium and hydrogen ion which would otherwise be secreted into the tubular urine to accompany non-reabsorbed anion.

It should be stressed that hydrogen ion in the proximal tubule may be excreted as titratable acid with titration of phosphate

$$(HPO_4^{2-}) + (H^+) \rightarrow (H_2PO_4^-)$$

whereas in the distal tubule, where the pH of the tubular fluid may be considerably lower, the hydrogen ion is buffered by creatinine ($pKa = 4.97$) and α ketobutyrate, rather than phosphate which has a pKa of 6.8.

Loading with potassium results in K^+ entering the renal tubular cells and displacing H^+ so that Na^+ which is absorbed from the luminal fluid is exchanged for K^+ fluid, which is secreted into the tubular lumen, rather than for H^+. Consequently the urine tends to be alkaline and there is loss of bicarbonate in the urine which may be inappropriate and result in a metabolic acidosis with a fall in extracellular fluid bicarbonate levels.

Question What happens to hydrogen ion in the cells in hypokalaemic alkalosis?

Answer 1. Decrease. Go on to **7.21**.
            2. Increase. Go on to **7.23**.

7.23   Your answer—Increase in H^+ intracellularly.

Good. You are correct. With hypokalaemia and potassium deficiency hydrogen ions enter the cells replacing the missing K^+ ions. This gives rise to a fall in H^+ concentration in the ECF and a resultant alkalosis resistant to all therapy other than replacement of the potassium deficit may be found.

When there is a loss of chloride ion e.g. due to vomiting, the bicarbonate *concentration* increases to fill the anion gap and there is a reduction of the extracellular volume giving rise to the descriptive terms *contraction alkalosis*. It is likely that a reduction of ECF volume causes an increase in the bicarbonate reabsorption threshold in the kidney. The reverse is true in cases of ECF volume expansion, where bicarbonate threshold falls and this results in a lowering of plasma bicarbonate levels i.e. dilution acidosis' occurs.

Elevation of $P\text{CO2}$ causes an increase in tubular reabsorption of HCO_3^- and a resultant fall in the quantity of bicarbonate excreted in the urine. The mechanism of this increase in tubular reabsorption of bicarbonate is as follows: the high $P\text{CO}_2$ causes an increase in intracellular (H^+)—you remember that from $P\text{CO}_2$ we can calculate dissolved CO_2 or H_2CO_3 by multiplying $P\text{CO}_2$ in mmHg by 0.03. Now $H_2CO_3 \rightleftharpoons H^+ + HCO_3^-$.

Thus the higher the $P\text{CO}_2$ the greater the H^+ concentration in the tubular cells. The excess H^+ will diffuse into the tubular urine and combine with HCO_3^- there, resulting in greater bicarbonate reabsorption. Consequently the urine has less bicarbonate in it and the patient has a higher plasma bicarbonate level than normal.

Let us go over this again

Contraction alkalosis norm is the term used to describe the situation which occurs when the ECF volume is reduced, for example by the use of diuretics which cause an increase in Na^+ and Cl^- excretion. As a consequence the volume of the ECF falls but the total amount of bicarbonate left in the ECF is unchanged; thus we have the same number of millimols of bicarbonate in a smaller volume of fluid i.e. the concentration of bicarbonate will rise. Thus there are more millimols per litre, although the total number of molecules of bicarbonate in the body is unchanged. It is a rise in bicarbonate *concentration* and *not* in *quantity* of bicarbonate. In practice it needs a considerable loss of ECF before there is an increase in bicarbonate concentration on purely 'contractional' grounds.

Dilution acidosis. When ECF is expanded with saline there is a fall in bicarbonate concentration due to the increase in ECF volume. This gives a 'dilution acidosis' in which the fall in bicarbonate concentration is supposedly due to mere dilution in saline. In practice because of the blood and bone buffers it is not usualy to find acidosis in patients with an expanded ECF. If an acidosis is found it is usually attributable either to other causes interfering with excretion of hydrogen ion—renal or respiratory—or there is a massive increase in ECF volume.

Question If the ECF is reduced in volume, what occurs?

Answer 1. Contraction alkalosis. Go on to **7.25**.
2. Expansion acidosis. Go on to **7.27**.

7.24   Your answer—1–3 mEq.
This is incorrect. You ought to read with more concentration. This is not a novel which you can speed read. It consists of facts you must learn. Learn **7.20** again.

7.25   Your answer—contraction alkalosis.
You are correct. Now let us look at some of the clinical disturbances of acid—base balance.

First of all it is possible to divide them into 4 categories: metabolic acidosis; respiratory acidosis; metabolic alkalosis; and respiratory alkalosis. Let us look at these in detail separately.

Respiratory acidosis   is characterized retention of carbon dioxide i.e. PCO_2 is elevated. The normal arterial PCO_2 is 40 mmHg and elevation of PCO_2 up to 100 mmHg can be seen in a variety of diseases. The diseases which cause respiratory acidosis may be acute or chronic (see Table 7.25(a) and (b)), and can be divided into those (a) in which the lung tissue itself is so damaged that CO_2 cannot diffuse out of the lung capillaries into the alveoli, as is seen in emphysema; and (b) in cases of obstruction of the airways as in status asthmaticus where gaseous exchange is impaired because gas cannot move normally into and out of the alveoli, the PCO_2 rises;

Table 7.25a   Causes of acute respiratory acidosis

All are causes of acute respiratory failure
Lung Disease
1. *Pneumonia*
2. *Pneumothorax*
3. *Pulmonary oedema*
4. Pulmonary embolus (massive)
Airways
1. Asthma
2. Foreign body
3. Aspiration of stomach contents
Neuromuscular
Self poisoning
Poliomyelitis
Polyneuritis
Hypokalaemia
Myaesthenia gravis

Learn this table and write it out with the book closed.

Table 7.25b Chronic respiratory acidosis

Lung Diseases
    Chronic obstruction airways disease
    (COPD in U.S.A.)
    Chronic interstitial pulmonary disease
    Ankylosing spondylitis and kyphosis
Neuromuscular
    Pickwickian syndrome
    Poliomyelitis, chronic state
    Amyotrophic lateral sclerosis

Learn these tables and write them out with the book closed.

Paralyses of the respiratory muscles, e.g. poliomylitis, muscular dystrophy, Guillaine-Barré syndrome Myaesthenia gravis, hypokalaemia, may be sufficient to prevent gaseous exchange because the thorax and diaphragms do not move adequately and so P_{CO_2} increases. Drugs—particularly morphine but also to a lesser extent pethidine may depress respiration centrally; Curare-like drugs which cause paralysis of the respiratory muscles are capable of causing respiratory alkalosis. Sleep is associated with diminished gaseous exchange and increase in P_{CO_2}. In all these conditions the metabolically produced CO_2 is unable to be excreted in the normal fashion, and so the P_{CO_2} rises and the pH falls according to the Henderson-Hasselbalch equation. Similarly a high P_{CO_2} causes an increase of urinary NH_3 and this is accompanied by loss of chloride in the urine.

This may be simplified into $H^+ = 24\ P_{CO_2}/HCO_3^-$ where $H^+ =$ nEq/l, $P_{CO_2} =$ mmHg, $HCO_3 =$ mmol/l,

$$CO_2 + H_2O \rightleftharpoons H_2CO_3 \rightleftharpoons H^+ + HCO_3^-$$

The increase in intracellular H^+ in the tubular cells of the kidney causes a rise in the H^+ being secreted into the tubular fluid for bicarbonate reabsorption, and consequently there is greater bicarbonate reabsorption. Similarly a high P_{CO_2} causes an increase of urinary NH_3 and this is accompanied by loss of chloride in the urine. Thus in respiratory acidosis there is a *rise* in plasma *bicarbonate*, with a *low pH* and a *high* P_{CO_2}. Read this paragraph again. You can differentially diagnose a high plasma bicarbonate: either it is due to respiratory acidosis with a low pH and a high P_{CO_2}; or it is due to a metabolic alkalosis, with a high pH and a low or normal P_{CO_2}; or a mixture of respiratory acidosis and metabolic alkalosis. You can correct for the P_{CO_2} effect on bicarbonate levels by using the 'Standard Bicarbonate' of Astrup and Siggard Anderson: in this the bicarbonate level is determined at a P_{CO_2} of 40 mm at 38°C and in fully oxygenated blood. The normal range is 21 to 25 mEq/l of plasma. If the level of Standard Bicarbonate is above 25 mEq/l there is a *metabolic* alkalosis; if it is below 21 mEq/l there is a *metabolic* acidosis. Similarly Astrup used the term base excess (1.2 × the deviation from the standard bicarbonate) to give a rapid measure of the degree of *metabolic* acidosis or alkalosis present. Metabolic alkalosis has Base Excess values greater than + 5 mEq/l; metabolic acidosis has Base Excess values of − 5 mEq/l or more. By and large there is little to be gained from using Standard Bicarbonate or Base Excess other than as a rough guide for therapy. The picture is complicated by the huge buffer capacity of the body and compensatory metabolic mechanisms which compensate for respiratory acidosis. Thus the changes in pH are limited by the huge buffering capacity of the reduced haemoglobin of the normal red cell.

Question A man has a P_{CO_2} of 80 mmHg, his arterial plasma pH is 7.25 and his bicarbonate is 38 mmol l^{-1}. What is your diagnosis?

Answer   1. Respiratory alkalosis. Go on to **7.28**.
          2. Respiratory acidosis. Go on to **7.30**.
          3. Metabolic alkalosis. Go on to **7.32**.

7.26   Your answer—a decrease in urinary ammonia loss.
    No. The increased intracellular pH associated with a high P_{CO_2} gives more H^+ production. This leads to an increase of urinary ammonia because the ammonia precursor enzymes are stimulated by chronic acidosis. Read **7.25** again and answer the question in **7.30**.

7.27   Your answer—expansion acidosis.
    You are wrong. How could a reduction in ECF volume cause any expansion of ECF? Use your head. Go back and reread **7.23**.

7.28   Your answer—respiratory alkalosis.
    No. Your answer is poor guesswork. First of all how can you pick alkalosis as an answer when the plasma pH is lower than normal? Read **7.25** again.

7.29   Your   answer—ammonia   excretion   is   increased.

You are correct. Treatment of respiratory acidosis depends on the cause. Mechanical obstruction to the airways, due to secretions in the trachea in the unconscious or paralysed patient can be removed by suction and tracheotomy. Status asthmaticus can usually be overcome by appropriate bronchodilator drugs and steroids. In obstructive airways disease, dead space may be reduced by tracheostomy. In the curare poisoned patient or poliomyelitic, use of mechanically aided respiration will cure the respiratory acidosis. In all these conditions the guide to therapeutic success in the return of $P\text{co}_2$ and pH of arterial blood to normal. Venous $P\text{co}_2$ is usually 6 mmHg greater than arterial but the blood sample must be taken without stasis i.e. no tourniquet. Makoff gives a good rule of thumb guide to changes in (H^+) and bicarbonate brought about by increasing $P\text{co}_2$ as follows.

In acute respiratory acidosis, the net effect is an increase in plasma hydrogen ion of 0.75 nEq/l for each mmHg elevation of $PaCO_2$. In Chronic Hypercapnia, there is an increase of 0.25 nEq/l in (H^+) for each mmHg of $PaCO_2$. *For every 3 mm $P\text{co}_2$ increase, plasma bicarbonate rises 1 mEq/l.* For moderate degrees of primary metabolic alkalosis ($HCO_3^- <$ 40 mEq/l), the $PaCO_2$ does not rise above 50 mmHg, so if the $PaCO_2$ is greater than 50 mm, then the patient is likely to have respiratory acidosis. If hypercapnia is known to be of brief duration and HCO_3^- is less than 25 mEq/l, then a cause for coexistent metabolic acidosis should be found. Read this again and learn it. Do not go on until you can be sure of writing it out correctly.

Question Do not look at the text above, but answer the question. In chronic hypercapnia how much does the hydrogen ion concentration increase for each mm of $PaCO_2$?

Answer 1. 0.25 mEq/1. Go on to **7.31**.
2. 1.0 mEq/1. Go on to **7.33**.

7.30   Your answer—respiratory acidosis.
You are correct. Now answer the next question.

Question In respiratory acidosis is there an increase or decrease in the urinary ammonia excretion?

Answer 1. Decrease. Go on to **7.83**.
2. Increase. Go on to **7.29**.

7.31   Your answer—0.25 mEq/litre.

You are correct. Now let us take a look at *Respiratory alkalosis.* Respiratory alkalosis is a condition in which the plasma pH is greater than 7.45 and the $PaCO_2$ lower than normal i.e. below 35 mmHg. (Pa means partial pressure in arterial blood.) Respiratory alkalosis has a variety of causes, the most frequent being psychogenic hyperventilation, a syndrome seen predominantly in young women who complain of symptoms of tetany—tingling in the fingers, toes and round the mouth, carpopedal spasm and light-headedness. The syndrome is usually one of the manifestations of hysteria. Hypocapnia, a lowered plasma PCO_2, is caused by a number of diseases in which there is hypoxia i.e. a low PO_2, and in an effort to remedy this the respiratory centre is stimulated to cause deeper and more rapid respiration. This results in a fall in PCO_2 while usually not restoring PO_2 to normal because CO_2 diffuses faster than O_2 through the alveolar—capillary barrier. A low PCO_2 associated with hypoxia, i.e. a low PO_2, is seen in alveolar—capillary block, pulmonary atelectasis and right—left shunts in congenital heart disease, and heart failure. In pulmonary emboli there is overbreathing with a low PCO_2 as a result. Similarly in lobar and broncho-pneumonia there is hyperventilation with a respiratory alkalosis being frequently found. A common cause of respiratory alkalosis is over-rapid or over-deep respiration of patients on mechanical respirators. Remember that the unconscious or curarised patient on a respirator has lost his protective mechanisms to regulate blood pH and PCO_2 and that frequent estimations of blood gases are necessary in these patients to provide the servo-mechanism for controlling speed and depth of respiration provided by the mechanical respirator. Salicylate intoxication can give respiratory alkalosis due to hyperventilation caused by stimulation of the respiratory centre, but there is often a metabolic acidosis component due to the ingestion of acetyl salicylic acid. Cirrhosis of the liver causes respiratory alkalosis. Staphylococcal pneumonia and Gram negative shock are causes of respiratory alkalosis due to stimulation of the respiratory centre by the bacterial toxins. Exercises, anaemia and learning to play wind instruments are causes of respiratory alkalosis. In diabetic ketosis, and lactic acidosis the respiratory alkalosis is complicated by the underlying metabolic acidosis.

It should be stressed that once the initial obvious overbreathing has taken place to initiate a respiratory alkalosis, maintenance of the lowered PCO_2 requires a less obvious effort which may be difficult to recognize clinically. Respiratory alkalosis is characterized clinically by:
1. Hyperventilation,
2. Tetany: in the mildest stages perioral tingling and tingling in the

hands and feet, followed later by carpopedal spasm, positive Chvostek and Trousseau's signs,

3. The urine becomes alkaline and has as a result phosphate precipitation, a sign known to all budding clarinetists and flautists who hyperventilate before they have mastered their instrument.

The physiology of the renal handling of bicarbonate and the buffering of hydrogen ion in the body is interesting. First of all, the fall in hydrogen ion concentration in the body because of the fall in $P\text{co}_2$ is buffered 1/3 by the blood buffers, particularly haemoglobin; and 2/3 by tissue buffers. There is also a rise in the organic acid levels in plasma, although these do not supply an important part of the buffering capacity.

Why does the plasma hydrogen ion level fall when $P\text{co}_2$ is lost in excess? Look at the formula $H^+ + HCO_3^- \rightarrow H_2CO_3 \rightarrow H_2O + CO_2$. Thus for every molecule of CO_2 breathed out in the lungs, one hydrogen ion is converted to water. Similarly plasma bicarbonate is lost in the process. Look at the formula. Hence plasma bicarbonate levels fall in hyperventilation, being lost in the proportion of one molecule of HCO_3^- for every molecule of CO_2 lost.

Question What is the commonest cause of acute respiratory alkalosis with tetany that you are likely to see in the accident (emergency) room in a young woman hitherto healthy?

Answer 1. Cirrhosis of the liver. Go on to **7.35**.
          2. Aspirin self poisoning. Go on to **7.37**.
          3. Hysterical hyperventilation. Go on to **7.39**.

7.32 Your answer—metabolic alkalosis.
      No. A $P\text{co}_2$ of 80 mm is very rarely seen in anything other than respiratory acidosis. Read **7.25** again.

7.33 Your answer—1.0 mEq/l.
      No. You are wrong. Read **7.29** again. Spend a good 5 minutes on this section.

7.34 Your answer—normal anion gap.
      No. The anion gap is $135 - 110 = 25$ mEq. Can you remember what is normal anion gap? Obviously you cannot or you would not have chosen this answer. Read **7.37** again please.

7.35   Your answer—cirrhosis of the liver.
   Although cirrhosis of the liver causes chronic respiratory alkalosis it rarely causes tetany and the question stressed 'acute' respiratory alkalosis. Cirrhosis of the liver is probably therefore the second choice and not the first. Read **7.31** again.

7.36   Your answer—raised anion gap acidosis.
   Good. You are correct. What are the causes of the 2 types of metabolic acidosis? Look at Table **7.36** and learn it.

Table 7.36   Differential diagnosis of metabolic acidosis (after Kaehny)

1. *Low or normal* anion gap (hyper-chloraemic)	2. *Increased* anion gap
1. *Gastro-intestinal loss of HCO_3^-* 　　Diarrhoea 　　Small-bowel or pancreatic 　　　drainage or fistula 　　Ureterosigmoidostomy, ileal 　　　loop conduit 　　Anion-exchange resins	1. *Increased acid production* 　　Diabetic ketoacidosis 　　Lactic acidosis 　　Alcoholic ketoacidosis 　　Inborn errors of metabolism
2. *Renal loss of HCO_3^-* 　　Renal tubular acidosis (RTA) 　　Diamox	2. *Ingestion of toxic substances* 　　Salicylate overdose 　　Paraldehyde poisoning 　　Methyl alcohol ingestion 　　Ethylene glycol ingestion
3. *Miscellaneous* 　　Dilutional acidosis 　　Addition of HCl or its 　　　congeners 　　Hyperalimentation acidosis	3. *Failure of acid excretion* 　　Acute renal failure 　　Chronic renal failure

   (a) *With a normal or reduced anion gap* i.e. hyperchloraemic acidosis.

1. Renal Tubular acidosis (RTA). This disease may be classified into (a) distal tubular (b) proximal tubular types and (c) incomplete (d) Hyporeninic hypoaldosteronism.
   Let us consider them in detail.

Proximal RTA is due to a defect in bicarbonate reabsorption in the proximal tubule, with a reduced $TmHCO_3$, so that bicarbonaturia occurs even when the plasma bicarbonate is low e.g. 15–20 mmol l^{-1} in normal persons. $TmHCO_3$ is not exceeded until plasma bicarbonate exceeds 25 mmol l^{-1} in normal health.

All types of RTA cause a hyperchloraemic acidosis with reduced or normal anion gap, but never an increased anion gap unless they have a complication such as uraemia, diabetic ketosis or lactic acidosis.

The **distal type** or **classical type** is associated with inability to maintain normal urine to blood hydrogen ion gradient which may be as high as 800 to one in a normal person i.e. pH of urine is 4.6, and pH of blood is 7.4. The cause of this inability is unknown. As a result of the RTA patients' inability to reduce the urine pH below 5.3 there is a constant decrease in NH_4^+ excretion and titratable acid. The lower the urine pH the greater the NH_4^- excretion and titratable acid (TA). Thus there is difficulty excreting the normal acid load and the pH of the plasma falls. This causes a fall in plasma bicarbonate.

$$H^+ + HCO_3^- \rightarrow H_2CO_3 \rightarrow H_2O + CO_2.$$

The CO_2 is blown off, and the plasma bicarbonate level is reduced. Thus the filtered load of bicarbonate is also lowered, and more chloride is reabsorbed with sodium in the proximal tubule, so that a hyperchloraemic metabolic acidosis results with a normal or low anion gap.

Distal RTA may be hereditary or may be caused by the following (Narins and Goldberg, 1977 classification):

1. Dysproteinuria: usually hyperglobulinaemia of any form such as biliary cirrhosis, Sjogren's syndrome, hyperglobulinaemic purpura, rheumatoid arthritis, cryoglobulinaemia, myeloma, etc.

2. Hypercalcaemia of any cause may interfere with acidification of urine and cause RTA.

3. Oedema forming states in which sodium absorption is so acid proximally that distal Na^+ ion delivery is minimal, inadequate for distal H^+/Na^+ exchange to permit adequate H^+ excretion.

4. Drugs: Amphotericin B, lithium and toluene damage renal function.

5. Renal Transplantation gives in 50 per cent of the patients distal RTA unmasked by giving an acid load. This is known as *incomplete RTA*.

6. Medullary Sponge Kidney, Hydronephrosis, Wilson's disease, sickle cell disease, all cause distal RTA. Pyelonephritis causes distal RTA.

Hypoaldosteronism diminishes distal H^+ secreting capacity and so permits the loss of bicarbonate. There is defective ammonia production and hyperkalaemia probably due to a rise in pH inside tubular cells.

In proximal RTA the patients can acidify their urine, but instead of reabsorbing all filtered bicarbonate when the plasma bicarbonate level is below 25 mmol l^{-1} as in the normal subject, they leak bicarbonate in the urine down to plasma levels of $15-20$ mmol l^{-1}, i.e. at least some of the nephrons have a $TmHCO_3$ lower than normal. This bicarbonate loss causes a fall in plasma bicarbonate. The daily loss of bicarbonate in the urine has to be replaced to prevent acidosis and can be given as sodium citrate. The amount of citrate required for any individual requires titration by trial and error, against the plasma bicarbonate level.

Proximal RTA. *In children* this is often a self-limiting disease but meanwhile requires therapy with sodium bicarbonate 10 mEq/kg. Some are associated with primary Fanconi syndrome—phosphaturia, bicarbonaturia, glycosuria, uric aciduria, amino aciduria. Presenting signs are often growth retardation and metabolic bone disease. Cystinosis is another cause of Fanconi syndrome, as is Tyrosinosis. Disorders of transport of fructose and galactose (due to deficiency of fructoaldotase and galactose uridyltransferase) also cause proximal RTA.

Adult forms of Proximal RTA.

(a) *Heavy metal*—poisoning by cadmium, lead, mercury, and copper. (Wilson's disease causes distal RTA.)

(b) Drugs—diamox, streptozotocin, outdated tetracycline, 6—mercaptopurine.

(c) Hormones—hyperparathyroidism described earlier.

(d) Dysproteinaemia—due to myloma dysglobulinaemia or, nephrotic syndrome—all cause a secondary Fanconi syndrome, as does Sjögren's syndrome myelomonocytic leukaemia.

(e) Renal Transplantation—in $\frac{1}{3}$ there is a *proximal* RTA syndrome. Remember $\frac{1}{2}$ have distal RTA post transplantation.

Question In distal RTA what is the abnormality?

Answer 1. Low $TmHCO_3$. Go on to **7.42**.

2. Inability to maintain the normal urine: plasma H^+ gradient. Go on to **7.40**.

7.37 Your answer—aspirin self poisoning.

Salicylates cause a mixed metabolic acidosis and a respiratory alkalosis. It is rare to see tetany in it. This should have been your second or third choice. Read **7.31** again.

7.38 Your answer—he has no acidosis.

This is a very poor guess. Since when is a pH of 7.25 in arterial plasma not an acidosis. Go back and read this chapter from 7.1 onwards. Do not day-dream.

7.39 Your answer—hysterical hyperventilation.

You are correct. In acute respiratory alkalosis there may be a high plasma lactate level. The cause of the rise in lactate level is possibly related to the increased lactate production in alkalotic tissues. In *chronic* hypocapnia i.e. lowered P_{CO_2}, on the other hand, there is no increase in plasma lactate concentration.

Metabolic acidosis. This is defined as an increased concentration of hydrogen ion in the ECF due to acids other than carbonic acid i.e. of metabolic cause. To understand what conditions may cause metabolic acidosis the anion gap should be examined. This is calculated by taking the plasma sodium concentration and subtracting from this the sum of plasma chloride and bicarbonate concentrations. Look at this example:

$$\Sigma \text{ cation } \{ \text{plasma Na}^+ \text{ (140 mEq)} = 140 \text{ mEq/l}$$

$$\Sigma \text{ anion } \{ \text{Cl (100)} + \text{HCO}_3 \text{ 28} = 128 \text{ mEq/l}$$

$$\text{Anion gap} = 140 - 128 = 12 \text{ mEq/l}$$

The normal anion gap in 10 ± 2 mEq/l. Metabolic acidosis can be thus divided into two groups—

1. With hyperchloraemia where the plasma chloride level is raised and thus the anion gap is normal or lowered. An example of this is in hyperparathyroidism which is associated with hyperchloraemic acidosis: typical findings are:

Plasma Na $= 140$ mEq/l
Plasma HCO$_3$ $= 15$ mEq/l   pH $= 7.20$.
Plasma Cl $= 113$ mEq/1

The anion gap is $140-128 = 12$ mEq/l i.e. a normal anion gap. There is hyperchloraemia, so the patient is said to be suffering from hyperchloraemic metabolic acidosis. The plasma electrolytes in chronic respiratory alkalosis are identical but in the latter the plasma arterial pH is alkaline. In hyperchloraemic metabolic *acidosis* it is acidic i.e. the pH is lower.

2. Increased anion gap e.g. normochloraemic metabolic acidosis is associated with an increased anion gap and a normal plasma chloride: typical figures of plasma electrolytes are as follows:

Plasma Na 140 mEq/l
Plasma Cl 100 mEq/l
Plasma HCO_3 15 mEq/l

Anion gap = $140 - 115 = 25$ mEq/l i.e. increased.

This is an increased anion gap and this immediately suggests another non-measured anion is present in excess quantity and is responsible for or associated with the metabolic acidosis.

Question In a patient there are the following biochemical findings:

Plasma pH (arterial)   7.25.
Plasma sodium   135.
Plasma chloride   100.
Plasma bicarbonate   10.

What type of acidosis is this?

Answer 1. Normal anion gap. Go on to **7.34**.
        2. Raised anion gap. Go on to **7.36**.
        3. He has no acidosis. Go on to **7.38**.

7.40 Your answer—inability to maintain the normal urine: plasma $[H^+]$ gradient.

Correct. Remember there is an incomplete form of distal renal tubular acidosis in which the patient is unable to acidify the urine but has no acidosis i.e. the plasma pH is normal. This can be made into a frank acidosis with an acid challenge.

Potassium depletion occurs *early* and *transiently* in the course of Proximal RTA when bicarbonaturia is prominent, but is otherwise not prominent. In contrast hypokalaemia is more frequent and constant in Distal RTA.

In acidosis, citrate reabsorption is enhanced in the proximal tubule, so that less is found in the urine. Citrate is a major chelator of calcium in the urine and so prevents calcium stone formation. This lack of urinary citrate is the cause of the high frequency of nephrocalcinosis and stone in *distal RTA*. In *Proximal RTA*, however, there is a defect in the reabsorption of citrate in the proximal tubule, so that the urine is rich in citrate which chelates calcium, and consequently, nephrocalcinosis and renal stone are *not* found in this type of RTA. Hyperchloraemic acidosis and hyperkalaemia result from damage to the juxta-glomerular apparatus, causing hyporeninism (low plasma renin) and in consequence, low plasma aldosterone levels. This is known as **Type IV Renal Tubular Acidosis**.

Distal RTA syndromes are seen in hydronephrosis, chronic pyelonephritis, hypercalcaemia and hypokalaemia. Ureterosigmoidostomy and ileal bladder cause RTA syndrome with hypokalaemic hyperchloraemic acidosis, due to the sodium and chloride ions in the urine being reabsorbed in the sigmoid in exchange for potassium and bicarbonate ions. The anion gap is normal in this condition which should be treated by a mixture of sodium and potassium citrates given orally and the dose adjusted according to the plasma bicarbonate and potassium levels.

Diamox (acetazolamide) causes a loss of bicarbonate, K and Na in the urine due to the inhibition of hydrogen ion production caused by inhibition of carbonic anhydrase. The patient develops a fall in plasma bicarbonate level, hypokalaemia and a metabolic acidosis.

Question A man has undergone reimplantation of his ureters into an ileal conduit, his bladder having been removed because of carcinoma. His plasma electrolyte study one year later shows:

Plasma Na	138 mEq/l.
Plasma K	2.8 mEq/l.
Plasma Cl	118 mEq/l.
Plasma HCO_3	12 mEq/l.

How would you correct his electrolytes?

Answer 1. Give him potassium citrate. Go on to **7.41**.
2. Give him sodium citrate. Go on to **7.43**.
3. Give him a mixture of sodium and potassium citrates. Go on to **7.44**.

7.41 Your answer—give him potassium citrate.

This is partly correct but unfortunately may cause hyperkalaemia. Read **7.40** again.

7.42   Your answer—a low $TmHCO_3$.

No. You are confusing proximal and distal RTA. Read **7.36** again and concentrate carefully. The material is loaded with facts. You cannot day-dream through it. If you want to, go and use a standard text. They are very good at permitting you to stare at the pages without the content getting into your brain or you ever knowing it is not getting in.

7.43   Your answer—sodium citrate.

This will not correct the hypokalaemia. Read **7.40** again.

7.44   Your answer—sodium and potassium citrate.

You are correct. Good.

Let us now look at the *Causes of a normal anion gap acidosis.* We will use Emmet and Narin's classifications. These can conveniently be divided into 2 classification groups:

(a) Those with normal or high serum K.

(b) Those with low serum K.

Let us look at them in detail.

(a) Normal or high serum K^+ normal anion gap metabolic acidosis.

1. *Hyperalimentation*—due to giving excess acid-generating material.
2. *Post hypocapnia*—discussed in text elsewhere.
3. *Dilution acidosis*—discussed in text elsewhere.
4. *Hypoaldosteronism.*
    1. Hyporeninism.
    2. Adrenal damage.
    3. Failure of tubular response to aldosterone.
5. *i.v. arginine or oral NH_4Cl therapy.*
6. *Early uraemic acidosis.*

(b) Low K normal anion gap metabolic acidosis.

1. RTA
    a. Distal, most commonly.
    b. Proximal, occasionally.
    c. Lack of phosphate buffer due to hypophataemia.
2. G.I. disorders.
    a. Diarrhoea.
    b. Pancreatic fistula.

3. Ureteral diversions.

a. Ureterosigmoidostomy (this has been discussed above) and ureteroileostomy.

In both these last conditions, bicarbonate and potassium are excreted into the urine from the gut in exchange for chloride and sodium, so that a hyperchloraemic hypokalaemic metabolic acidosis ensues.

Now let us look at acidosis with an **increased anion gap**. In metabolic acidosis with an increased anion gap there is usually an increase in the level of organic acids in the plasma. Thus we see metabolic acidosis with an increased anion gap in:

i. Diabetic ketosis where the extra anion is hydroxybutyric acid. The clinical features are the deep, acidotic (Kussmaul) respiration, severe reduction in ECF volume due to loss of sodium in vomit and excretion of sodium ion with hydroxybutyric acid because it has a very low pKa (2.8) and thus in the blood and urine is virtually all in the form of the organic salt β-hydroxybutyrate rather than in the form of the acid. Remember that at a pH above the pKa more than 50 per cent is in the salt form and at a pH below the pKa the acid is the predominant form. Accompanying β-hydroxybutyric acid in the plasma is acetone which is readily detected by the physician's nose. The smell of acetone in the presence of acidotic respiration is diagnostic of diabetic ketosis unless the patient is using acetone either as a nail polish remover or as an elastic dressing remover. Lactic acidosis frequently complicates diabetic ketoacidosis and causes a further increase in anion gap.

ii. Renal failure. In severe renal failure there is an increase in salts of organic acids in the blood—among them being creatinine, guanidino-succinic acid, guanidiono-proprionic acid; and sulphates. In addition the ability of the kidney to excrete hydrogen ion is diminished: because of the reduction in functioning renal mass there is a reduction in the maximum possible ammonia production and so a fall in ammonium ion excretion. $NH_3 + H^+ \rightarrow NH_4^+$. Similarly with a fall in GFR the amounts of filtered phosphate and creatinine are reduced, although the urine pH may fall as low as 4.6. This results in a fall in titratable acid excretion: together with the fall in NH_4^+ excretion and in titratable acid, the ability to excrete the normally produced 50–70 mEq of H^+ that are formed in the body each day is grossly impaired. Some of this hydrogen ion is titrated by the bone salts, particularly calcium carbonate in the bone lattice, with resultant reduction in the mineral content of the bone. In addition there is often a bicarbonate wasting tubular defect where bicarbonate reabsorption is incomplete despite a fall in the plasma bicarbonate level to well below 25 mmol l^{-1}. It has been suggested by Muldowney that excessive levels of parathyroid hormone, such as are found in hyperparathyroidism secondary to renal failure are responsible for this bicarbonate leak.

Acute infusions of PTH impair proximal sodium reabsorption and in the distal tubule chloride reabsorption exceeds that of bicarbonate so that bicarbonaturia occurs.

Question What makes up the increased anion gap in diabetic ketoacidosis?

Answer 1. Phenols. Go on to **7.46**.
2. Lactic acids. Go on to **7.48**.
3. β-hydroxybutyric acid. Go on to **7.50**.

7.45 Your answer—lactate is metabolized in muscle and the red cell.

No. Lactate is formed in muscle and the red cell; it is metabolized elsewhere. Read **7.50** carefully again and find the correct answer.

7.46 Your answer—phenols.

You are incorrect. This is a guess. Read **7.44** again but more carefully this time.

7.47 Your answer—liver and kidney.

You are correct. Let us now look at the prognosis of lactic acidosis.

The prognosis of lactic acidosis is poor. Most die frequently of underlying diseases. Let us use Relman's (1978) classification of causes of **lactic acidosis**.

1. *Tissue hypoxia*—poor tissue perfusion due to shock, sepsis, asphyxia, acute left ventricular failure.
2. *Drugs:*
    1. Ethyl alcohol often with non-diabetic ketoacidosis, or an ethanol binge, in a chronic alcoholic.
    2. Phenformin—now banned in the U.S. Most dangerous where there is impaired renal function causing high levels of blood lactate.
    3. Methanol—breakdown products of its metabolism stimulate glycolysis and lactate accumulation.
    4. Salicylates—uncouple oxidative phosphorylation in the mitochondria and stimulate glycolysis.

5. Ethylene glycol, dithiazanine, streptozotocin, isoniazide, nitro-prusside.
6. Fructose and sorbitol cause lactic acidosis because of rapid con-version of fructose to fructose 1 phosphate depleting hepatic ATP, and so inhibiting hepatic metabolism of lactate.
3. *Adrenaline* (Epinephrine): enhances glycogenolysis and causes tissue anoxia by vasoconstriction.
4. *Liver failure*: failure of liver to metabolize lactate.
5. *Neoplastic* disease.
6. *Pulmonary embolism*: in presence of shock and anoxaemia.
7. *Sepsis caused* tissue anoxia.
8. *Diabetes Mellitus*: a frequent concommittant either with phenformin or with ketoacidosis. A higher incidence of lactic acidosis is found in renal failure.
9. *Idiopathic* or unknown cause.
10. *Congenital*—due to abnormalities in gluconeogenesis or oxidation of pyruvate and caused by enzymatic defects.

Symptoms These are few symptoms ascribable to lactic acidosis *per se*, other than those of acidosis i.e. dyspnea, lassitude, weakness, fatigue, stupor or coma.

Diagnosis The diagnosis is suggested by a large anion gap in an acidotic patient in whom there is no hyperglycaemia, or uraemia, history of acute alcoholism or aspirin ingestion. Phenformin ingestion in a diabetic would be suggestive of lactic acidosis but not conclusive.

Therapy This depends on the cause and the extent of the lactic acidosis. Shock with levels of lactic acid of greater than 8 mEq/l is most frequently fatal. However in all cases the therapeutic approach should be:

(1) Correct the acidosis with i.v. sodium bicarbonate
(2) Increase tissue oxygenation. This may require blood transfusion, oxygen via respirator and Isuprel or L-dopamine infusions.
(3) Cessation of phenformin therapy.
(4) Antibiotics of appropriate type in cases of septic shock.
(5) Insulin in diabetic hyperglycaemia and *diabetic* ketoacidosis complicated by lactic acidosis.
(6) In *uraemic* lactic acidosis, haemodialysis rather than functional dialysis is the better choice because acetate is present in the haemo-dialysate whereas lactate is most frequently found in peritoneal dialysis solutions. It is obviously wiser to attempt connection of acidosis and

uraemia without increasing lactate concentration as is frequent in peritoneal dialysis.

Question If the lactate level is 12 mEq/l, what is the likelihood of a fatal outcome?

Answer 1. Very likely fatal. Go on to **7.51**.
2. Will recover. Go on to **7.52**.

7.48 Your answer—lactic acid.
You are partially correct in that lactic acidosis complicates diabetic ketoacidosis frequently. This is not the answer you should have given on the text of **7.46**. Go back and read **7.46** again.

7.49 Your answer—lactate is metabolized in brain and skin.
You are wrong. You are confusing metabolism with production of lactate. Read **7.50** again but concentrate carefully this time.

7.50 Your answer—β-hydroxybutyric acid.
Correct. Let us now deal with lactic acidosis.

Lactic acidosis. In lactic acidosis the normal metabolism of lactate is impaired usually due to the presence of tissue hypoxia. Lactate is the end of the line for carbohydrate metabolism. Lactic acid is normally present in the peripheral blood. In arterial blood, in health, its concentration is less than 1.5 mEq/litre. In venous blood it is normally higher depending on whether there was stasis and muscular exercise in the muscles from which the veins drain. Thus if venous lactic acid levels are measured the arm from which the blood is drawn should be at rest and without stasis i.e. without a tourniquet. Venous lactate levels are up to 4.5 mEq/litre. Lactic acidosis is a serious and often fatal condition. It is due to pyruvate being converted to lactate instead of being metabolized to CO_2 and water. The formation of lactic acid is due to reduction of pyruvate acid to lactic acid. Lactic acid can only be converted to pyruvate and hence oxidized but this is a slow process. Lactic acid levels may increase in the plasma due to (1) Increase production of lactic acid due to breakdown of glycogen (2) Decrease in conversion of lactic acid to pyruvate. Lactate is metabolized by liver and kidney. Lactate is produced by 1. red cells (responsible for $\frac{1}{4} - \frac{1}{2}$ lactate production, 2. exercising muscle, 3. brain, 4. skin.

Question By what organs is lactate metabolized?

Answer 1. Muscle and red cell. Go on to **7.45**.
2. Liver and kidney. Go on to **7.47**.
3. Brain and skin. Go on to **7.49**.

7.51 Your answer—it is very likely going to be fatal.
Correct.

Oral ingestion of acids. Ammonium chloride is given by mouth in the Wrong and Davies test for maximal urinary acidification in a dose of 0.1 g per kg body weight. This causes a metabolic acidosis over a period of about 5–8 hours, with a fall in plasma pH and bicarbonate transiently, because NH_4Cl is metabolically equivalent to the ingestion of HCl. Salicylate intoxication may result from therapy in rheumatic fever or rheumatoid arthritis, or in cases of attempted suicide. It causes a complicated series of changes in acid–base metabolism—(1) respiratory alkalosis due to the direct effect of salicylate on the respiratory centre; (2) metabolic acidosis caused by several metabolic effects including glycogenolysis, uncoupling of oxidative metabolism, hyperglycaemia, ketosis and increased production of organic acids. There is a bicarbonate diuresis and enhanced potassium excretion. Thus there may be a metabolic acidosis, or a respiratory alkalosis or a mixed picture with respiratory alkalosis and metabolic acidosis in competition, the final pH depending on which is stronger.

A typical example of diabetic ketoacidosis giving an increased anion gap is as follows—

Sodium	132 mEq/l
Chloride	85 mEq/l
Bicarbonate	11 mmol/l

Anion gap $= (132 + \quad) - (85 + 11) = 132 - 96 = 36\ mEq/l$.
This increase in the anion gap is caused by β-hydroxybutyric acid. When there is a chronic metabolic acidosis there is an accompanying hyperventilation with a resultant fall in P_{CO_2} of approximately 1 mmHg for every mEq fall in bicarbonate. The hyperventilation may continue for several hours after the metabolic acidosis has been corrected by bicarbonate and give rise to a severe respiratory alkalosis.

This is due to the lag in the fall of the CSF pH which remains elevated for several hours after the plasma pH has returned to normal.

Question In a patient with diabetic ketoacidosis there is a large anion gap of 25 mEq/l, but lactate levels are not increased. What is the substance most likely to be responsible for most of the increased anion gap?

Answer 1. Acetone. Go on to **7.54**.
　　　　2. β-hydroxybutyric acid. Go on to **7.53**.
　　　　3. Acetoacetic acid. Go on to **7.55**.

7.52　Your answer—the patient will recover.

No, it is unlikely that he will recover. This is clearly stated in the paragraph **7.47**. You cannot be concentrating properly. Go back and learn the contents of **7.47** again.

7.53　Your answer—β-hydroxybutyric acid.

You are correct. The therapy of a metabolic acidosis should be divided into two parts: (1) Treatment of the underlying disorder: i.e. therapy of diabetic ketosis with ECF replacement therapy and insulin, dialysis for uraemia. (2) Correction of the acidosis. This can be achieved using sodium bicarbonate after ascertaining that there is no hypocalcaemia in the case of a chronic acidosis. In the presence of hypocalcaemia this must first be corrected to prevent a further reduction in ionized calcium levels caused by the increasing plasma pH: a further fall in already low ionized calcium levels may cause tetany; this may be so severe as to include generalized convulsions which in the chronically acidotic patient with osteomalacia or osteoporosis may result in fractured long bones. Thus, if there is hypocalcaemia this should be treated by intravenous 10 per cent calcium gluconate 10 ml given i.v. over a period of 5 minutes. If hypocalcaemia is absent or once it has been treated, therapy of severe metabolic acidosis is by intravenous sodium bicarbonate. It is convenient to work with molar strength sodium bicarbonate because there is no need for calculation: 1 mEq is present in each ml of molar $NaHCO_3$. In the U.S.A. the commonly used $NaHCO_3$ solution contains 45 mEq per ampoule. The patient should have plasma pH and P_{CO_2} measured and then be given 100 mEq—200 mEq of Na HCO_3 i.v. slowly over 5 minutes and then half an hour after the end of the injection further measurements of pH and P_{CO_2} are made. To assume that the dose of bicarbonate to be given is equal to base deficit $\times \frac{1}{2}$ body weight expressed as mEq is misleading. In many patients it may prove to be inadequate, particularly if they have lactic acidosis and are resistant to large or even massive doses of sodium bicarbonate. In any case the safest way is to try it in small doses, i.e.

give 100 or 200 mEq at first, even if the theoretical dose is 400 mEq. Wait $\frac{1}{2}$ to 1 hour, *repeat the blood gases* and recalculate the dose needed then give a further dose of 100–200 mEq of sodium if the pH is not within the safe range.

This bio-servo mechanism is essential if you are to save patients by avoiding dogmatic decisions. Always be conservative and monitor your patient's responses. Do not use these doses in the presence of renal failure, for the sodium in the $NaHCO_3$ cannot be excreted and so is potentially able to expand the ECF resulting in right heart failure or hypertension and left heart failure. Remember the aim of intravenous bicarbonate administration is not to restore the plasma pH to normal limits, but to restore it so that (1) it is in a safe range i.e. above 7.2; (2) the acidosis is so mild that the respiratory drive is reduced. This may be a very slow process. (3) That if hyperkalaemia is present then the plasma pH should rise by at least 0.2 units to reduce the K^+ in plasma by 2 mEq/ litre. Of course in many patients correction of the acidosis with the initial 100–200 mmol of $NaHCO_3$ will be adequate to correct the base deficit and restore plasma pH to normal limits. In cases where control with sodium bicarbonate is difficult due to renal failure not permitting adequate therapy with massive doses of $NaHCO_3$, because of its sodium content, then dialysis will usually correct a metabolic acidosis smoothly. Remember that in all electrolyte disturbances which are proving difficult in practice to treat by intravenous injection of electrolyte solutions of varying composition satisfactory results can be obtained with the minimum of difficulty and the maximum of safety by the use of peritoneal dialysis or haemodialysis. Both these techniques are particularly valuable in their smoothness of correction of difficult electrolyte problems.

Question If you have a very complex electrolyte problem—say lactic acidosis with hypercalcaemia and hyperkalaemia in a patient with acute renal failure, how would you treat it?

Answer 1. Dialysis. Go on to **7.56.**
2. Various i.v. electrolytes. Go on to **7.58**.

7.54 Your answer—acetone.

You are incorrect. Acetone is not the cause. Read **7.51** again carefully. You are not concentrating. This time either concentrate and drive out your distractions or give up your attempt to learn for the present. Do not fool yourself. In a standard format book you can day-dream, but not in this type of book.

7.55 Your answer—aceto-acetic acid.

You are partly correct but β-hydroxybutyric acid is more important. Read **7.51** again, and do not day dream.

7.56 Your answer—dialysis.

You are correct.

Metabolic alkalosis has received much attention in the past 20 years with a great deal of benefit to patients suffering from the various diseases which cause metabolic alkalosis. First a definition: metabolic alkalosis is a condition where there is an actual decrease in hydrogen ion concentration in the plasma due to either excessive loss of hydrogen ion from the body or actual addition of base or hydroxyl ion or its equivalent to the body. Biochemically it is characterized by a plasma arterial pH above 7.45, an increased plasma bicarbonate above 30 mEq/l, and a normal or slightly increased P_{CO_2} always less than 60 mmHg. There is a fall in plasma chloride pari passu with the rise in plasma bicarbonate. In respiratory alkalosis P_{CO_2} is of course lower than normal. In chronic lung disease plasma bicarbonate is elevated but so is the P_{CO_2} (often above 60 mmHg), and the plasma pH is either normal or low.

Metabolic Alkalosis is characterized by an alkaline pH i.e. higher than 7.45, high P_{CO_2} and raised (HCO_3^-) in the plasma. There is a fall in plasma chloride pari passu unless there is an increase in plasma sodium for other reasons, or of unmeasured anions such as lactate or acetoacetate.

Physiology of respiratory compensatory response to metabolic alkalosis. There is a reduced rate of alveolar ventilation in metabolic

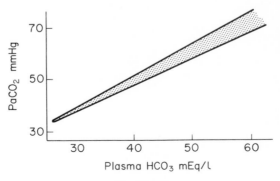

Fig. 7.56I

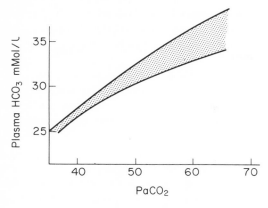

Fig. 7.56II

alkalosis due to a fall in hydrogen ion concentration causing a reduction in chemical neuroreceptor stimulated messages to the medulla controlling alveolar ventilation. The degree of hypercapnia (i.e. P_{CO_2} elevation) is directly related to the amount of the alkalosis as expressed by the plasma bicarbonate. Look at Fig. 7.56I. If K deficiency is present, there is either less compensation or none. This is because K deficiency induces an intracellular acidosis, and this counteracts the intracellular alkalosis induced by the metabolic alkalosis.

How can we tell if there is a coexisting respiratory acidosis with a metabolic alkalosis? By looking at a histogram of the relationship between blood HCO_3^- and $PaCO_3$. If the plasma bicarbonate is greater than can be accounted for by the P_{CO_2}, then there is a metabolic component. Look at Fig. 7.56II. If at $PaCO_2$ of 50 mm the bicarbonate is 45 mmol l^{-1} then a metabolic component is present.

Question A man has the following biochemical values.

Plasma $PaCO_2$ 40 mmHg.
Plasma pH   7.62.
Plasma HCO_3 50 mmol l^{-1}

What is his acid–base disorder?

Answer 1. Respiratory alkalosis. Go on to **7.57**.
2. Respiratory acidosis. Go on to **7.59**.
3. Metabolic alkalosis. Go on to **7.60**.
4. Metabolic acidosis. Go on to **7.61**.

7.57 Your answer—respiratory alkalosis.

If you were correct then you would expect the P_{CO_2} to be low. It is not. Read **7.56** again and choose the correct answer.

7.58 Your answer—various electrolyte solutions i.v.

You may be right but in practical terms if you have an artificial kidney available or peritonial dialysis facilities, it is easier to correct the complex abnormalities by dialysis than by custom built i.v. electrolyte cocktails. Go on to **7.56**.

7.59 Your answer—respiratory acidosis.

You have made a poor guess. How on earth do you take an alkalaemia and say it is an acidosis? Also the P_{CO_2} is not high enough for a respiratory acidosis. Guessing is not the aim of learning. Read more carefully **7.56** and concentrate. Use your head. You are not reading a novel.

7.60 Your answer—metabolic alkalosis.

You are correct. Good. If respiratory acidosis and metabolic alkalosis coexist then the P_{CO_2} is greater and hypoxaemia more severe.

What are the causes of metabolic alkalosis?

1. Loss of hydrogen ion through the G.I. tract: Pyloric stenosis; vomiting of any cause; aspiration of stomach and an upper small bowel.

2. Mineralocorticoid excess. Cushings syndrome has as a major biochemical disturbance a hypokalaemic alkalosis due to loss of excessive amounts of hydrogen ion and potassium in the urine. These changes are due to large amounts of circulating corticosteroids causing an increased distal tubular reabsorption of sodium and consequently an increased exchange for (H^+) and (K^+). Chloride is normally absorbed distally with sodium, but with the ion for ion exchange of sodium ion for H^+ and K^+, chloride cannot be absorbed at this site and consequently chloride ion is lost in large amounts in the urine. This results in a state of chloride depletion, with a metabolic hypokalaemic alkalosis. Correction requires both potassium salts and chloride to be supplied, potassium ion alone or chloride ion alone will not correct the hypokalaemic alkalosis. The hypokalaemia of Cushings syndrome is most pronounced in Cushings syndrome caused by adventitious secretion of corticosteroids from bronchial carcinomata. Aldosteronism, primary or secondary, and licquorice intoxication are causes of metabolic alkalosis with hypokalaemia. In Bartter's syndrome there is a hypokalaemia metabolic alkalosis with normal blood pressure and hyperreninaemia and hyperaldosteronaemia, mediated in part by prostaglandins.

Question A man with Cushing's Syndrome has a severe hypokalaemic alkalosis (serum K $= 1.8$ mEq/l). What is the most likely cause?

Answer 1. Prednisone therapy. Go on to **7.62**.
         2. Adrenal hyperplasia. Go on to **7.64**.
         3. Carcinoma of the bronchus. Go on to **7.66**.

7.61 Your answer—metabolic acidosis.
    Your answer is a guess. How can you pick an acidosis when the pH is alkaline? Read **7.56** again. This time concentrate. Do not just day-dream and stare at the pages.

7.62 Your answer—prednisone therapy.
    You are wrong. Predisone induced Cushing's Syndrome has minimal mineralocosticoid effects, so the K level should be normal. Read **7.60** again.

7.63 Your answer—intracellular hydrogen ion concentration is increased.
    You are correct. Good. Let us now consider.

1. Alkalosis after hypercapnia. When a patient becomes hypercapnic chronically, there is a chloride diuresis and the plasma bicarbonate level increases as more bicarbonate is reabsorbed renally. A state of chloride depletion occurs, with a depressed plasma chloride level and an increased plasma bicarbonate level. When the cause of the hypercapnia has been effectively treated and the $P\text{co}_2$ has returned to normal, a chloride depletion alkalosis still persists. This will continue until repletion of chloride has been carried out by administration of say, ammonium chloride. Always be wary of using potassium chloride. There is evidence that at local concentrations of greater than 7 mEq/litre, potassium chloride causes ulceration of the mucosa of the small intestine into which it comes in contact. 'Slow K' was designed to overcome this, but the occasional patient gets intestinal ulceration with stricture and/or perforation despite the resin-embedded slow release form of slow K.

2. Milk–alkali syndrome. Excessive intake of antacids such as sodium bicarbonate, magnesium hydroxide and calcium carbonate together with large amounts of milk, is responsible for the development of the milk–

alkali syndrome which may be complicated by severe alkalosis, hyper-calcaemia, metastatic calcification with or without nephrocalcinosis.

Excessive quantities of sodium bicarbonate taken orally may exceed the kidneys' ability to excrete bicarbonate and thus may cause a severe alkalosis.

If there is a metabolic alkalosis, hypoventilation is a compensatory mechanism of limited value, and there is a rise in $P\text{CO}_2$ which rarely rises above 60 mmHg.

Hypercalcaemia and metastatic calcification including nephrocalcinosis results from the high calcium intake.

Question The following biochemical findings were in a patient with nephrocalcinosis.

Serum calcium	13.5 mg/100 ml.
Serum HCO_3^-	45 mol/l.
Arterial pH	7.58.
$PaCO_2$	50 mmHg.

Answer 1. Renal failure. Go on to **7.68**.
2. Hypercalcaemia. Go on to **7.69**.
3. Milk–alkali syndrome. Go on to **7.71**.

7.64 Your answer—adrenal hyperplasia.
No, in **7.60** this point is discussed. Read **7.60** again and pay more attention this time. You have missed a point which was described.

7.65 Your answer—hydrogen ion intracellular concentration is un-changed.
You may be partly correct. The many patients on diuretics there is no overall potassium deficit. However, if there is a potassium deficiency then hydrogen ion will enter the cells to replace potassium. Read **7.66** again.

7.66 Your answer—carcinoma of the bronchus.
You are correct. Good.

3. Diuretics. Loss of potassium from the body may be caused by per-sistent use of diuretics without replacement of losses of potassium. Some of the potassium loss is due to the development of a state of hyperaldo-steronism which causes sodium reabsorption and potassium loss from the distal tubule and collecting ducts. Chloride depletion in diarrhoea of any cause, including the rare congenital chloridorrhoea or due to potassium and chloride secreting papilloma of the colon and rectum, causes an increase in plasma bicarbonate levels due to the lack of availability of chloride ion in the distal tubule for reabsorption with sodium; thus bicarbonate is reabsorbed instead and consequently the plasma bicarbonate rises. Loss of potassium ion from the body causes K depletion and loss of hydrogen ion in exchange for sodium in the distal tubule with absolute loss of excessive amounts of hydrogen ion. Similarly in the cells there is a rise in hydrogen ion concentration due to H^+ replacing intracellular K, and there is consequently a fall in the extracellular fluid hydrogen ion concentration. There are thus both renal and cellular losses of hydrogen ion. Replacement with extracellular fluid in the form of sodium chloride solution with potassium ion added should correct both the alkalosis and the potassium and chloride depletion.

Question What may happen to intracellular hydrogen ion concentration in a patient given thiazide diuretics for many months without potassium supplement?

Answer 1. (H^+) Increases. Go on to **7.63**.
 2. No change. Go on to **7.65**.
 3. (H^+) Decreases. Go on to **7.67**.

7.67 Your answer—intracellular hydrogen ion decreases.
  No. This is the wrong answer. You should pick the correct answer after reading **7.66** more carefully. Do not guess and do not day-dream.

7.68 Your answer—renal failure.
  No. You have no evidence for this. Please do not make ridiculous guesses. Read **7.63** again.

7.69 Your answer—hypercalcaemia.
  You are partially correct. However hypercalcaemia is not the only abnormality. There is also a metabolic alkalosis. Hypercalcaemia, metabolic alkalosis and nephrocalcinosis are found in milk–alkali syndrome. Read **7.63** again, and this time concentrate on the text. Do not dream your way through it.

7.70 Your answer—metabolic alkalosis.
  No. The P_{CO_2} is the clue. Read **7.71** again.

7.71 Your answer—milk–alkali syndrome.

Good. You are correct. Treatment of metabolic alkalosis is divided into (1) treatment of the primary disease; (2) treatment of the metabolic alkalosis itself. Now treatment of the primary disease is itself outside the scope of this book—therapy of Cushings syndrome, aldosteronism, excessive diuretics and so on being dealt with in general textbooks of medicine. Potassium and chloride depletion must be corrected: chloride can be given as sodium chloride where no heart, kidney, liver disease or hypoproteinaemia are present. If any contraindication to sodium administration is found, then the chloride can be given in the form of ammonium chloride which is cheap, given orally, and found in most pharmacies or intravenously as arginine hydrochloride. Never forget that an ordinary diet will often correct K^+ and Cl^- deficits in a few days. If the electrolyte disturbance is complicated or difficult to correct, a dialysis can be used to correct the abnormalities as a last resort. Now let us look at some odd pieces of information it is advantageous to know.

Measurement of intracellular pH. Intracellular pH differs from extracellular pH: although extracellular pH can readily be measured by taking the plasma and putting it through a pH electrode, intracellular pH is more difficult to measure. There are two methods of measuring intracellular pH:

(1) Use of direct means. This involves use of microelectrodes which are small enough to be inserted into the cells. This method involves damaging the cell when the electrode passes into the wall, and in any case the actual term intracellular pH is probably a will-o'-the-wisp, for the intracellular subcellular particles are not a homogeneous single structure, but each has its own particular structure and physiology and is likely to have a hydrogen ion concentration characteristic for its enzymatic requirements. Nevertheless microelectrode potentials give an intracellular pH in the region of 6 to 7.1 depending on the tissue and type of electrode used. There is no doubt that much ink has been spilled in a vain attempt to explain a difference of a few tenths of a pH unit in the results when the meaning of intracellular pH is itself a blanket term of no clear meaning.

(2) Use of indirect means. By using a weak acid such as DMO (dimethyl oxazolidinedione) the distribution of DMO in its ionized form across the cell is dependent on the pH inside the cell. This is an indirect method and again even if the answer given is accurate it gives an impression of the mean pH inside the cell and not of its individual subcellular components such as nuclei, mitochondria, Golgi apparatus etc. Most valves of intra-cellular pH by this method are higher than by the direct method and are in the range of pH 6.9 to 7.1.

It is time to go over some of the major acid–base disturbances again. Let us now look at some examples of blood gas/pH results:

pH	7.29
P_{CO_2}	80 mmHg
P_{O_2}	56 mmHg
HCO_3	38 mmol/l^{-1}

This picture is of respiratory acidosis such as can be seen in status asthmaticus. Look at the low P_{O_2}, the acidosis, the HCO_3^- and the very high P_{CO_2}. Nothing else can give this picture. Let us look at the next example:

pH	7.55
P_{CO_2}	17 mmHg
P_{O_2}	80 mmHg

This is an example of respiratory alkalosis. Note the low P_{CO_2} and high pH. This is an example of a metabolic alkalosis. The next example is easy to identify.

pH	7.55
P_{CO_2}	45 mmHg
HCO_3	38 mmol/l^{-1}

This is an example of metabolic alkalosis. Note the alkalotic pH, very slight increase in P_{CO_2} and high bicarbonate level.

Finally, the next example is fairly easy to identify.

pH	7.20
P_{CO_2}	23 mmHg
HCO_3	13 mmol/l^{-1}

Note the low pH and low bicarbonate and low $P\text{CO}_2$. This is an example of a metabolic acidosis. Frequently there is a respiratory attempt to compensate for a metabolic acidosis or alkalosis, but in clinical practice the primary abnormality is rarely in doubt.

Question Now cover up the example and look at the acid–base findings in a patient.

Plasma pH	7.55.
$Pa\text{CO}_2$	15 mmHg.
$Pa\text{O}_2$	80 mmHg.

Answer 1. Metabolic alkalosis. Go on to **7.70**.
2. Respiratory alkalosis. Go on to **7.72**.
3. Normal. Go on to **7.73**.

7.72 Your answer—respiratory alkalosis.
Good. Now look at the 3 statements below and choose the correct answer.

1. $(\text{H}^+) = 24 \dfrac{P\text{CO}_2}{(\text{HCO}_3^-)}$

2. Haemoglobin is a more important buffer than the plasma proteins.
3. In proximal RTA the urine pH is always above pH 5.3.

Now choose the correct answer.

Answer 1. All statements are true. Go on to **7.74**.
2. All statements are false. Go on to **7.75**.
3. Statement 1 is true, 2 and 3 are false. Go on to **7.76**.
4. Statement 2 is true, 1 and 3 false. Go on to **7.77**.
5. Statement 3 is true, 1 and 2 false. Go on to **7.78**.
6. Statement 1 is false, 2 and 3 true. Go on to **7.79**.
7. Statement 2 is false, 1 and 3 true. Go on to **7.80**.
8. Statement 3 is false, 1 and 2 are true. Go on to **7.81**.

7.73 Your answer—normal.
This is a poor guess. How can a pH of 7.55 be normal? Can a $Pa\text{CO}_2$ of 15 be normal? No. So read **7.71** again.

7.74 Your answer—all the statements are true.
If that is your answer, you have not understood RTA at all. Read **7.36** again and go on from there.

7.75   Your answer—all the statements are false.

No. The first 2 statements are true. You should read from **7.1** to **7.36** and then answer the question in **7.72** correctly.

7.76   Your answer—only statement 1 is true.

You are wrong. Statement 2 is true. Start reading **7.1** through **7.36** and then answer the question in **7.72** correctly.

7.77   Your answer—only statement 1 is true.

No. You have forgotten that statement 2 is true. Go back and read **7.1** through **7.36** again, and then answer the question in **7.72** correctly.

7.78   Your answer—statement 3 is true.

You are quite wrong. Read this chapter again in its entirety.

7.79   Your answer—statement 1 is false.

No. You are wrong. Read the entire chapter again. Then answer the question in **7.72** again.

7.80   Your answer—statement 2 is false.

No. You are wrong. Read through the chapter again.

7.81   Your answer—statement 3 is false.

You are correct. Before leaving this subject I would recommend the following reading:

The most useful up-to-date book is that edited by Brenner B. H. and Stein J. (1978) *Acid Base and Potassium Homeostasis*. Churchill Livingstone, London.

Chapters particularly recommended are:

The Renal Acidosis R. Narins

Lactic Acidosis, A. Relman

Metabolic Alkalosis, A. Sebastian, H. Hulter and F. C. Rector

Acid Base Disorders of Respiratory Origin, J. J. Cohen and N. E. Madia

There are also frequent articles in *Nephron, Kidney International, Renal Physiology* and *Am. J. Physiology* embracing these subjects. *Contributions to Nephrology*, a series by Karger has very up-to-date original articles which are highly recommended.

7.82   Your answer—none.

This is a remarkable guess and shows clear evidence of your day-dreaming your way through this book. Stop it. Read **7.20** again and then choose the correct answer.

7.83   Your answer—decrease.

Your are correct. Read **7.25** again.

Chapter 8
Parenteral Nutrition

8.1   One of the problems confronting the doctor in hospital is how to manage a patient by use of parenteral feeding i.e. intravenous nutrition in a patient who is incapable of taking food by mouth, due to operations on the gastro-intestinal tract, burns, sepsis including peritonitis, obstruction of the oesophagus etc. Intravenous nutrition is referred to as 'hyperalimentation' a word which is both unsuitable and incorrect in the majority of cases, but which is in widespread use and therefore must be learned. Intravenous nutrition is by definition the supply of the foodstuffs needed for the maintenance of health via the veins rather than the gastro-intestinal tract, and includes not only carbohydrates, fats and amino acids, but also the minerals and vitamins necessary for normal health. There is now abundant evidence that it is possible to supply by the intravenous route everything needed to keep the patient in a satisfactory state of nutrition. To do so we must supply the following constituents:

1. Calories. These can be supplied either as carbohydrate which supplies 4 calories per gram, or as fat which supplies 9 calories per gram: protein contains 4 calories per gram: alcohol supplies 7 calories per gram. It will therefore be seen that gram for gram fat supplies the most calories; alcohol comes next and then carbohydrate and protein at the lower end of the scale. For obvious reasons, in countries where alcoholism is a problem, there is a tendency to eschew the use of this drug in i.v. feeding. Protein can be removed at once from the list. Intravenous protein is restricted to the following:

1. Whole blood: this is given if there is blood loss.

2. Plasma: this is given in cases of loss of plasma proteins, as in burns; or in patients who have low serum protein levels due to inability to synthetize adequate amounts due to lack of absorption as in stratorrhoea or starvation; due to liver disease where the liver is unable to synthesize albumen as in the case of hepatic cirrhosis; or where there is protein loss as in burns, protein losing enteropathy and nephrotic syndromes.

3. Salt-free Plasma albumin. This is costly and is indicated where there is a need for salt free replacement of plasma albumin: this is neces-

sary in conditions of sodium retention with hyperaldosteronism such as in cirrhosis and nephrotic syndrome.

Protein should only be given intravenously to *replenish* plasma protein levels. You must *not* give protein intravenously to maintain nutrition because protein given intravenously is very inefficient in supplying the necessary amino-acids needed for tissue protein building. It has been calculated that i.v. protein is only 1/2000 as efficient as the appropriate amino-acids. Let us consider amino-acids as bricks and protein as the completed house. If you want to build a house it is more efficient to buy the correct sized bricks which you can assemble with mortar to build the walls rather than to buy a complete house and then break it up into its constituent building materials and then maybe you do not have the requisite number of suitable sized bricks: maybe they are too few or of the wrong size and you find this out after the work of breaking down the walls. Amino-acids are the building bricks of protein: they have to be present in the correct concentration, with appropriate composition of the necessary amino-acids, to form the appropriate protein needed by the body in the tissue under consideration. Read this again. There is no sense in giving plasma or albumen when we need amino-acids. Proteins take days to break down totally to amino-acids. Also amino-acids are cheaper than plasma albumin, and do not carry serum hepatitis (hepatitis B), whereas pool plasma certainly does. Thus intravenous amino-acids are in daily use for intravenous nutrition: they are the building blocks of the proteins. We will return to consider them later, but first we must go back to the major energy suppliers—carbohydrates and fat.

Question If a patient has to be fed parenterally for a prolonged period and has a normal serum albumin level, would you give him his daily nitrogen requirements as intravenous albumin, plasma, or amino-acids?

Answer 1. Intravenous albumin. Go on to **8.3**.
2. Plasma. Go on to **8.4**.
3. Amino-acids. Go on to **8.5**.

8.2 Your answer—200 calories.
No. In 2 litres of 5 per cent dextrose there are 100 g of dextrose. How many calories is that? Is it enough to sustain life? Read **8.5** again.

8.3 Your answer—i.v. albumin.
No. If you give i.v. albumin, you have to wait for the protein to be

broken down into its individual amino-acids before it can be used for making new protein. This may take 10 or more days, during which the patient becomes progressively malnourished and may not have enough amino-acids of appropriate type in circulaton to enable synthesis of the immuno-globulins essential in the overcoming of infection. Read **8.1** again.

8.4   Your answer—plasma.

This is not correct. To obtain amino-acids for the synthesis of immunoglobulins and other proteins essential for the body's defense against infection one cannot wait for several days until the plasma is broken down. You need amino-acids, so give amino-acids. Read **8.1** again.

8.5   Your answer—amino-acids.

Good. Do not forget that you need amino-acids in the right composition at the right time and with adequate calories to synthesize the proteins used in healing and in the fight against infection, so that is why they should always be given in parenteral nutrition. Remember that Blackburn has demonstrated a very clear protein sparing effect when i.v. amino-acids are given intravenously, even when the calorie intake is less than desired, i.e. under circumstances which would normally result in massive loss of protein to provide the calories for day to day bodily needs.

The carbohydrates supply us with 4 calories for each gram. They are a major source of calories, and of those carbohydrates in common use, glucose and fructose are the most popular. Glucose requires insulin for its immediate metabolism, whereas this is not the immediate limiting factor with fructose. On the other hand fructose may induce lactic acidosis. Glucose can be given in 5 per cent solution. One litre of 5 per cent glucose has 50 g of glucose or only 200 calories in it. 10 per cent glucose is irritant to veins as is 20 per cent but nevertheless they may need to be given. A litre of 20 per cent dextrose (virtually the same thing as glucose which is dextrose monochydrate) contains 800 calories. A healthy man resting in bed needs 1400 calories. A burned patient may need 4000 calories a day. So the carbohydrate supply of calories is obviously quite inadequate if there is any limit on the quantity of fluid that may be given.

8.5   **Question** How many calories a day can you get from giving a patient 2 litres of 5 per cent dextrose i.v. daily?

Answer   1. 200 calories. Go on to **8.2**.
2. 400 calories. Go on to **8.7**.

8.6   Your answer—soya bean oil.

Correct. Fortunately not only is Intralipid ® safe but it also contains over 50 per cent linoleic and linoleinic acids, the essential fatty acids without which we develop dermatitis. It is essential to remember that Intralipid is emulsified with egg yolk lecithin, and therefore will occasionally cause reactions in some people who are sensitive to eggs. Because it is an emulsion *it must not be mixed with anything at all* before it gets into the vein. Remember this, never put anything in the bottle of Intralipid. The substance is so bland that it can be given through tiny peripheral veins on the back of the hand. The supplying of calories has to be simultaneous with the supply of amino-acids if they are to be utilized for anabolic purposes rather than excreted in the urine. If the calories source is given in one 12 hour period and the amino-acid source is given in the next 12 hour period, then much of the amino-acids infused cannot be utilized and are excreted. Let us pause for a minute and consider why do we need to supply calories every day parenterally, for example after an operation. Are there enough stores of energy to tide a patient over a couple of weeks? The answer is that it depends on the patient's state of nutrition and obesity, but it is worth while looking at the facts in Table 8.1 for a 70 kg man of average nutrition.

Substance	Amount (g)	Calories	Comment
CHO	200	1,800	Lasts a few hours.
Fat	8500	76,500	Use alone associated with ketosis. Enough for 30 days calories supply post-operatively.
Protein	2000	8,000	Alone adequate for calorie supply of 4 days.

The carbohydrate stores are principally present as liver glycogen and they are lost in a few hours. Protein stores last a few days before the readily mobilized protein pool is burned up for calories. Fat stores last the longest. It is obvious that in the septic burned patient with a hypercatabolic state where 4000 or more calories are being used per day, that calories have to be supplied intravenously, together with amino-acids, or the patient will lose body mass rapidly (both fat and muscle) and soon die. Weight loss due to utilization of protein in muscle to supply calories may amount to a kg each day, if calories and amino-acids are not supplied. If you have a patient who is on i.v. nutrition and you want to know approximately how much protein he is breaking down per day there is a simple technique for working this out. Let us take an example first of a patient with normal renal function. Measure the urea nitrogen excreted in the urine: say 10 g per day. (28 g out of every 60 g of urea are nitrogen, urea is $CO(NH_2)_2$ and the molar weight of urea is 60, of which nitrogen is 28.)

But on the average there is 1 g of N in every 6.25 g of tissue protein, so that the amount of protein broken down is $10 \times 6.25 = 62.5$ g.

If you want to use urea rather than urea N then because $28/60 \times 6.25 = 2.92$, multiply the total daily urea excretion by 2.92 i.e. $2.92 \times 20 \cong 60$ g.

However this does not take into account 2 factors:

1. Urea broken down in the gut. This amounts to 1.5 g N per day in the absence of disease of the gastro-intestinal tract. 1.5 g of N is equivalent to 6.25×1.5 g of protein $= 9.46$ of protein.

2. Nitrogen in the urine which is not in the form of urea i.e. uric acid, creatinine, amino acids etc. This is usually about 7.5 per cent of the total N output so that to correct the urea figure we should multiply it by $100/100-92.5$ i.e. 108. Thus the total protein breakdown from urine N losses is $2.92 \times 1.08 \times 20 = 63.0$ g/day. If we add in the 9.5 g of protein equivalent to urea broken down in the gut in the supposed intestinal loss we get a total of 72 g of protein catabolized. To keep the patient in nitrogen balance on parenteral nutrition we have to supply the amino-acids in the correct composition and in amount equivalent to $72/6.25$ g of nitrogen per day, together with adequate calories i.e. 11.52 g of amino-acid N per day. If there is associated renal damage we take the urine urea as described and *in addition* the blood urea nitrogen rise each 24 hours is measured. If there is no increase in blood urea nitrogen levels, then there is no need to change the urine calculation. If there is a rise in the BUN levels, then the body weight is measured and from this, in the absence of oedema or dehydration the total body water is obtained: total body water is about 60 per cent of body weight. A 70 kg man has 42 kg of water in his body. Now urea is distributed throughout body water, so that the blood urea rise is equivalent to adding urea to the entire body water. Let us take an example. BUN rises in 24 hours from 100 to 110 mg per 100 ml in a 65 kg man. Daily increment in BUN $= 10$ mg/100 ml $= 100$ mg/l. Total body water $= 65 \times 0.6$ litres $= 39.0$ litres, therefore total urea nitrogen added to body water in 24 hours $= 39 \times 100$ mg $= 3.9$ g.

This is urea which resulted from protein metabolism but has been added to the body water and not excreted in the urine therefore the amount of protein this represents = 3.9 × 6.25 = 24.4 g protein. This must be *added* on to the protein breakdown derived from the urinary urea figures.

Question How much protein is equivalent to 1 g of nitrogen?

Answer 1. 2.92 g. Go on to **8.8**.
           2. 6.25 g. Go on to **8.11**.

8.7   Your answer—400 calories.

Good. Now 400 calories is even less than the Nazis gave their Auschwitz prisoners, so you can see that next time you go round the intensive care unit and see patients getting only two litres of dextrose a day as a 5 per cent solution, then you can realize that they are being starved to death by their incompetent physicians. You need at least 1400 calories if you are lying quietly in bed, but if you are post-operative you need from 2500 to 3500 or more calories a day to keep up with calories being used. The infected pyrexial hypercatabolic patient may need considerably more. The burned patient needs at least 4000 calories, depending on the amount and depth of the burns and the degree of infection. So go round and save lives by pointing out what calorie intake is needed.

Of course there is very frequently some renal damage in patients who require intravenous or parenteral nutrition which causes limitation of their fluid intake, so their calorie requirements cannot be met satisfactorily from carbohydrates alone. For this purpose intravenous fats are convenient in that they are the most concentrated energy source we have. Remember fats have 9 calories for each gram. The most suitable fats for intravenous use at the moment of writing are soya bean oil emulsified with egg phospholipid. This is known commercially as Intralipid, and is manufactured by Vitrum in Sweden, and marketed by Cutter Lab. U.S.A. It should be understood that they are not absolutely safe: they very rarely cause anaemia and sometimes thrombocytopenia, but there are particularly few side effects if less than 2 g/kg/day are infused. The solutions are 10 per cent and 20 per cent.

One litre of 20 per cent contains 200 g of fat and is too much for the average 70 kg patient. On the other hand, 1 litre of 10 per cent contains 100 g of fat i.e. 1.4 g/kg/day for a 70 kg man and supplies 900 calories. If fluid volume has to be restricted then 500 ml of 20 per cent Intralipid will supply 900 calories in the minimum of fluid.

Question Is Intralipid made from cotton seed oil or soya bean oil?

Answer 1. Soya bean. Go on to **8.6**.
2. Cotton seed. Go on to **8.9**.

8.8 Your answer—2.92 g.
You are confusing the conversion factor for urea which is 28/60×
6.25. Read **8.9** again very carefully. It is not easy reading and not designed
for the day-dreamer.

8.9 Your answer—cotton seed oil.
No. This is incorrect. The cotton seed oil lipid preparations on the
whole were not too safe and in many countries are not used at all. In the
U.S.A. the FDA forbids the use of all but Intralipid, which is mainly Soya
bean oil.

8.10 Your answer—egg protein.
You are correct. There is no point in giving aminio-acids without a
simultaneous source of calories. This can be as a mixture aminosol—fructose—ethanol, with ethanol having not only a calorie providing role, but
also a specific nitrogen sparing action and giving the patient a sense of
well being. Remember not to give alcohol at a rate of greater than 10 g/hour
or the patient might become intoxicated. Both alcohol and fructose can
cause lactic acidosis (see Chapter 7). The amount of calories which should
be given should be 200 times the number of grams of nitrogen being given,
at least i.e. for a daily intake of 15 g of N as amino-acids one should provide
at least 3000 calories. When N is given intravenously as amino-acids, and
provided renal function is normal then potassium must be supplied because
when nitrogen is laid down as protein K is taken up by the cell in a ratio
of 1 mEq K per g of nitrogen: therefore whenever amino-acids are supplied
care should be taken to administer potassium simultaneously *provided
no renal damage is present*. At the same time as the i.v. amino-acids and
fructose are being given it is wise to drip in Intralipid, the soya bean oil
fat emulsion, simultaneously. This not only supplies calories and has
a well defined protein sparing effect but appears to prevent thrombophlebitis to a certain extent as well.
Electrolytes need to be supplied to keep the patient in balance. Prolonged intravenous feeding leads to magnesium and phosphate depletion,
so it is wise to have the electrolyte composition of urine and drainage
fluid examined daily for sodium, potassium, calcium, *magnesium* and

phosphate. If there is no phosphate in the infusion and prolonged i.v. feeding is being undertaken when phosphate depletion may occur. Remember magnesium and phosphate depletion may be present on admission to hospital in alcoholics. To prevent this phosphate may need to be supplied i.v. as a buffered sterile solution of $NaHPO_4/NaH_2PO_4$ at pH of 7.4 but this has to be prepared in advance and kept in stock. Large quantities should not be given for they may cause hypocalcaemia. This has already been discussed in the chapter on calcium metabolism.

Question What two elements may be deficient in alcoholics on admission to hospital?

Answer 1. Sodium and potassium. Go on to **8.12**.
             2. Magnesium and phosphorus. Go on to **8.14**.

8.11   Your answer—6.25 g.
        Good. You are correct. The composition of the amino-acid mixture needed is of great importance. Firstly, only L amino-acids are utilizable in man (with the exception possibly of methionine where the D form may be utilizable). Secondly, the essential amino-acids must be supplied in composition close to that in egg reference protein, but this varies from person to person.

Essential amino-acids are not synthesizable in the body. Look at Table 8.11 for a list of essential amino-acids.

Table 8.11   Essential amino-acids

1. Leucine	4. Methionine	7. Valine
2. Isoleucin	5. Tryptophane	8. Threonine
3. Lysine	6. Histidine	9. L Phenylalanine

Histidine is an essential amino-acid in normal persons and in uraemic patients. Arginine appears to be an essential amino-acid in infancy and in patients getting parenteral nutrition. *Non-essential amino-acids can be synthetized in the body*, but conditions of synthesis vary, so that it is advisable to add glycine protein and serum in all mixtures.
        The ratio between essential amino-acids and the total amino-acids is known as the E/T ratio. For egg and human milk, (these being standard reference proteins of the FAO, and ideal in their amino-acid composition) the E/T ratio is 3.2. It is advisable to use an intravenous amino-acid

mixture with an amino-acid composition and E/T ratio close to that of an egg. Aminosol is particularly close (E/T ratio 3.01), but there are various proprietary brands available in each country. Remember that amino-acid mixtures are frequently casein or beef serum hydrolysates and as such may contain electrolytes such as Na and K. However, totally synthetic L amino-acid mixtures are now available and some are electrolyte free. These must be taken into account in patients with electrolyte or renal function disturbances.

Question Which common foodstuff has the ideal amino-acid composition?

Answer 1. Meat. Go on to **8.13**.
2. Eggs. Go on to **8.10**.

8.12 Your answer—sodium and potassium.
They may be depleted if the patient has had a prolonged alcoholic gastritis or pancreatitis. This was not discussed in **8.10**. Something else was. Read **8.10** again please.

8.13 Your answer—meat.
You are not correct. Meat has a less desirable composition than eggs. I am excluding human meat of course, but expect that few of my readers will be cannibalistic in tendency.

8.14 Your answer—Mg and P.
Correct. The route of prolonged intravenous feeding is a problem. It is usual to use a plastic catheter inserted into a peripheral vein and keep it in use in the same place for one or two weeks and then move to another side as soon as the first signs of thrombophlebitis appear— tenderness and reddening of the infusion site. Alternatively, if it is known that intravenous feeding is necessary for a prolonged period of time i.e. when virtually all the small intestines have been resected, then it is wise to follow the method introduced by Scribner of using an artificial arterio-venous fistula, such as Cimino Brescia fistula, for needling repeatedly with a small needle for each day's infusion; or a special subclavian shunt with a silastic catheter implanted subcutaneously.

In prolonged infusion all the water soluble vitamins have to be given intravenously, or intramuscularly. It is particularly necessary to supply the daily requirements of the following vitamins: Vitamin B_1 (aneurine or thiamine), Nicotinamide, Vitamin B_6 (pyridoxine), Pantothenic acid,

Biutin, Vitamin B_{12}, Vitamin C (ascorbic acid) and Folic acid. The fat soluble vitamins A, D and K can be given intramuscularly as a depot preparation if intravenous feeding is prolonged. Otherwise it is doubtful whether they need to be given for short courses of i.v. nutrition of one or two weeks due to the considerable liver stores of fat soluble vitamins. The exact doses do not need to be remembered. They are to be found in the Appendix should you need them. Do not lumber your mind with unnecessary facts; there are sufficient important things to learn and remember.

Alcohol which has a calorie value of 7 cal/g has not only a valuable protein sparing effect, but has also a mild euphoric effect which many patients enjoy. To avoid actual intoxication with alcohol the average patient should not get more than 10 g/hour. Do not give alcohol to alcoholics. Beware of the possibility of causing lactic acidosis with it and monitor lactate levels daily when it is used. Because infusion of amino-acids increases the rate of disappearance of alcohol from the blood stream it is wise to give alcohol and amino-acids together—indeed there is commercially available an amino-acid fructose—ethanol mixture (Aminosol ethanol fructose). Remember that fructose and ethanol can both precipitate lactic acidosis. Blood gases and lactate levels need monitoring daily when they are used for i.v. feeding.

In renal failure if parenteral nutrition has to be undertaken e.g. after major gastro-intestinal surgery, then intravenous nutrition has to be modified in the following manner:

1. The nitrogen supplied as essential amino-acids should be the minimum to prevent under-nutrition.

2. The sodium and potassium content of the amino-acid solutions must be taken into account. Aminosol for example contains about 100 mEq of sodium per litre. The aim in renal failure is not to change the internal environment, and clearly the addition of 100 mEq of sodium is a serious problem, which you will see shortly can only be got over by frequent dialysis. Alternatively electrolyte free L amino acid solutions can be used i.e. FreAmine.

3. The volumes of water provided in intravenous nutrition regimens are considerably more than the 500 ml/day and urine losses and drainage which are necessary to maintain body water homeostasis in the oliguric patient.

This problem can be solved by daily haemodialysis; or failing that, dialysis on a daily or alternate daily schedule. It is thus possible to maintain fluid and electrolyte balance despite the necessity of giving 2 litres or more of intravenous fluids daily containing considerable quantities of sodium ion, chloride ion and potassium ion. Obviously the conditions of the dialysis have to be tailored to the special requirements of the patient who receives i.v. nutrition i.e. adequate ultra-filtration to remove the excess fluid, and potassium concentration in the dialysis fluid appropriate to the parenteral potassium load.

Question If the patient post-operatively has renal failure and is oliguric how would you manage him if he needs 3 litres of i.v. fluids a day in excess of his calculated fluid requirements including drains and suction?

Answer   1. Don't give him the fluid. Go on to **8.16**.
2. Dialyse him daily to remove fluid. Go on to **8.18**.

8.15   Your answer—2.8 litres.
     You are correct. *Blood* is given in 25–50 per cent burns according to the formula 1 per cent of the patient's blood volume for each 1 per cent of skin burned, instead of plasma. Now total blood volume in ml = wt in kg $\times$ 75; therefore in a man weighing 70 kg the blood volume is 5250 ml and if he has 30 per cent burns he should get 30 per cent of 5250 i.e. 1750 ml of blood instead of plasma. This should be given partly in the second period i.e. at 4–8 hours after the burn and partly in the sixth period i.e. at 24 to 36 hours after the burn. Blood has to be given because of red cell destruction in the burned tissue; on all burns over 10 per cent of the body surface, anaemia is sufficiently severe to warrant blood transfusion, but relatively smaller milder burns of 10–25 per cent of body surface need the blood transfusion only in the period from the 24th to 36th hour.

Water and electrolytes: the burned patient needs parenteral fluid if vomiting occurs, which is common in extensive burns, i.e. over 35 per cent of body surface. The amount to be given is 60–100 ml/hour, with solutions containing adequate sodium and potassium to maintain the electrolyte loss in the urine. After the first day plasma is given to maintain serum albumin levels within the normal range and appropriate electrolytes should be given to replace losses of electrolytes in the urine and maintain a central venous pressure of 12–14 cm. It is equally necessary to measure acid–base balance and correct any metabolic acidosis which may occur, with appropriate doses of bicarbonate. Renal failure should be treated with doses of frusemide (Lasix) sufficiently large i.e. up to

2 g/day to maintain a reasonable diuresis of 1 to 2 litres/day. There is little evidence that frusemide will prevent renal failure, but the increased urine volume is useful in permitting a greater intravenous fluid intake. If parenteral nutrition is required then the burned patient requires massive replacement intravenously of amino-acids to replace the protein lost by hypercatabolism and in the exudate of the burn which is equivalent to a negative nitrogen balance of 10 g/day. Similar the exudate sodium loss may be 19 to 20 times as great as urinary loss. The average nitrogen loss to be replaced is equivalent to 1.2 g of protein/kg body weight and 60 cal/kg body weight. If the burned patient is not vomiting, a diet of egg, milk, glucose or caloreen, (a glucose polymer) and peanut oil should be given as a slow drip over 24 hours so that a total intake of over 4000 calories and 85 g of protein is achieved. In the event of renal failure being present with a creatinine clearance of less than 10 ml/minute, then haemodialysis should be undertaken whenever the blood urea rises to over 200 mg/100 ml (BUN 100 mg/100 ml), or if there are signs of excessive expansion of the ECF with a CVP (central venous pressure) in excess of 16 mm, hypertension, left ventricular failure or pleural effusion; severe acidosis, hyponatraemia or hyperkalaemia are all corrected safely with haemodialysis. Remember that in burns as with other hypercatabolic renal failures adequate calorie and nitrogen replacement can be safely undertaken if daily, or alternate daily haemodialysis is undertaken. This is the key to prevention of severe emaciation unmasked when the oedema of the burn disappears. In addition, because two of the major causes of death in the burned patient with renal damage are hyperkalaemia and septicaemia it is advisable to prevent at least the first with haemodialysis, and the institution of haemodialysis on a daily, or alternate daily, basis may also facilitate the safer administration of nephrotoxic and ototoxic amino-glycoside antibiotics even when there are no facilities to determine their plasma levels.

In summary then, the burned patient represents all the major problems in fluid, electrolyte, plasma protein and red cell loss with complicating gastro-intestinal and hypercatabolic problems. He requires about 60 cal/kg body weight and 1.2 g of protein per kg body weight per day. Vigorous replacement of plasma and blood is needed in the first 36 hours, together with careful monitoring of the electrolyte and water status and the acid–base status; and appropriate replacement of losses in urine, gastric drainage. If there is a weighing bed available then an attempt should be made to maintain the weight of the patient constant by appropriate i.v. fluid, but relatively few burns units are ideally equipped.

Question In a burned patient who does not die of septicaemia, what is the leading cause of sudden death?

Answer 1. Hyperkalaemia. Go on to **8.19**.
2. Pulmonary embolism. Go on to **8.21**.

8.16 Your answer—do not give him the fluid.

This is quite wrong unless you have no dialysis facilities at all. Sorry, but you are not concentrating when you read. This point was discussed in **8.14**. Read it again.

8.17 Your answer—1 litre.

No. You should multiply the patient's weight by the percentage burned and give half of the result in ml every 4 hours. Read **8.18** again.

8.18 Dialyse daily.

You are correct. Good. The burned patient is a particular problem. It is best to consider the fluid and electrolyte balance in the burned patient as being of two groups.

1. The early loss of protein containing fluid.
2. The problem of supplying adequate calories and nitrogen in a patient who commonly has as a complicating factor mild or severe, acute renal failure.

In practical terms when dealing with fluid loss in a burned patient it is wise to use the rule of 9s. This is a useful approximation which you should learn. Look at the diagram. This tells the extent of the burn, excluding mere erythema.

Plasma. In the burned patient there is a tremendous loss of plasma and also destruction of red cells, which must be taken into account. We do this by using the formula of Muir and Barclay which is as follows:

Every 4 hours for the first 12 hours the patient is given:

$$\frac{\text{ml of plasma}}{\text{every 4 hours}} = \frac{\text{Total area of burn per cent} \times \text{weight in kg}}{2}$$

The patient's central venous pressure, urine volume/ hour, haematocrit and haemoglobin are monitored. If the condition of the patient is satisfactory then at the end of the first 4 hours the dose of plasma is repeated; this is also the rule at the end of the second 4 hour period. If he has deteriorated, appropriate increase in parenteral fluid is indicated. 12 hours after the burn the patient is given the same amount of plasma

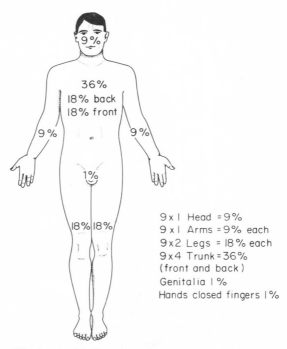

9%

36%
18% back
18% front

9%   9%

1%

18% 18%

9 x 1 Head = 9%
9 x 1 Arms = 9% each
9 x 2 Legs = 18% each
9 x 4 Trunk = 36%
(front and back)
Genitalia 1%
Hands closed fingers 1%

The hand with fingers adducted
and extended is 1%

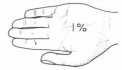

1%

Fig. 8.18

at 6 hourly intervals until 24 hours after the burn, when the same volume
is given at a further 12 hourly interval.

Question A man weighs 70 kg and has 80 per cent burns, what volume
of plasma should he be given every 4 hours for the first 12 hours?

Answer 1. 1 litre. Go on to **8.17**.
            2. 2.8 litres. Go on to **8.15**.

8.19   Your answer—hyperkalaemia.

Good. Now let us look at the statements below and then choose the appropriate answer.

Statement 1. 400 calories a day is adequate for the post-operative patient.

Statement 2. L amino acids are utilized by the body.

Statement 3. Intralipid should not be mixed with anything.

Answers 1. Statement 1 is true, 2 and 3 false. Go on to **8.20**.
2. Only statement 2 is true. Go on to **8.22**.
3. Only statement 3 is true. Go on to **8.23**.
4. Only statement 1 is false. Go on to **8.24**.
5. Only statement 2 is false. Go on to **8.25**.
6. Only statement 3 is false. Go on to **8.26**.
7. All statements are true. Go on to **8.27**.
8. All statements are false. Go on to **8.28**.

8.20. Your answer—statement 1 is true.
No. You are wrong, so start at **8.1** again

8.21 Your answer—pulmonary embolism.
It may occur, but it was not discussed in **8.15**. Go back and find what you have missed while day-dreaming.

8.22 Statement 2 is true.
No. You are wrong. Read on from **8.6**.

8.23 Statement 3 is true.
So is statement 2. Read again from **8.11**.

8.24 Statement 1 is false.
You are correct. I recommend Lee's *Parenteral Nutrition* and Allen and Lee's Clinical Guide to *Intravenous Nutrition* published by Blackwell Scientific Publications, Oxford, for further reading.

8.25 Statement 2 is false.
No. Start at **8.1** again.

8.26 Your answer—Statement 3 is false.
You are wrong. Read from **8.1** again.

8.27   All are true.

No. Start at **8.1** again.

8.28   All are false.

No. You are correct about the first. Start at **8.11** and read through this short chapter. You need the information in it.

Appendix

Vitamins required to be added to i.v. feeding in adults and children.

Thiamine—adults 1.2 mg/day (0.02 mg/kg);
infants 0.5 mg/1000 cal (0.05 mg/kg).

Riboflavine—adults 1.8 mg/day (0.03 mg/kg);
infants 0.1 mg/kg up to age 18.

Niacin—nicotinic acid ⎫ 6.6 mg/1000 cals.
nicotinamide ⎭

Pyridoxine (B_6)—adults 2 mg (0.03 mg/kg);
Infants 2 mg (0.1 mg/kg).

Folic acid—Minimal requirements: Adults—3 μg/kg;
infants 20 μg/kg.

Vitamin B_{12} derivatives: an injection of 1 mg i.v. or s.c. every 6 months is more than adequate.

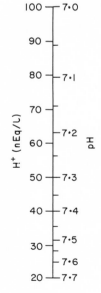

Appendix I

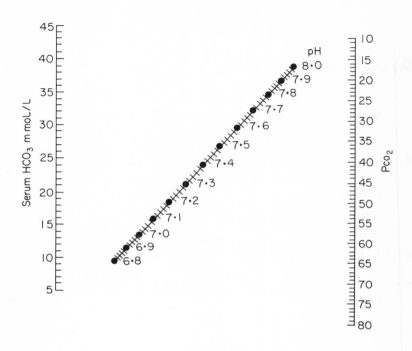

Appendix II

Pantothenic acid—adults 0.2 mg/kg;
                    infants 1.0 mg/kg.
Biotin—adults 5 μg/kg;
          infants 30 μg/kg.
Ascorbic acid (Vitamin C)—Adults 30 mg (0.5 mg/kg);
                            Infants 15–30 mg (3 mg/kg).
Vitamin A—adults 10 μg/kg;
              infants 100 μg/kg.
Vitamin D—adults 2.5 μg (0.04 μg/kg);
              infants 2.5 μg/kg.
Tocopherol is present in intra lipid 0.1 mg/g of fat.

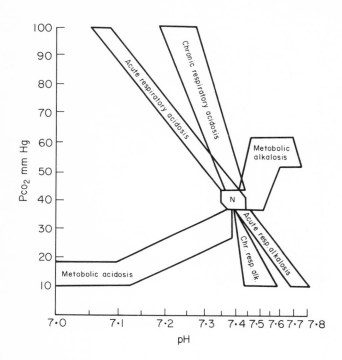

This diagram is reproduced by courtesy of Dr. E. Goldberger from *Electro-lyte and Acid–Base Disorders*. 5th edition, Lea and Febiger, Philadelphia.

Appendix III

Mineral requirements for an adult:

Ca	5 mMol
Mg	1.5 mMol
Fe	50 μMol
Mn	40 μMol
Zn	20 μMol
Cn	5 μMol
F	50 μMol
I	1 μMol

Appendix IV

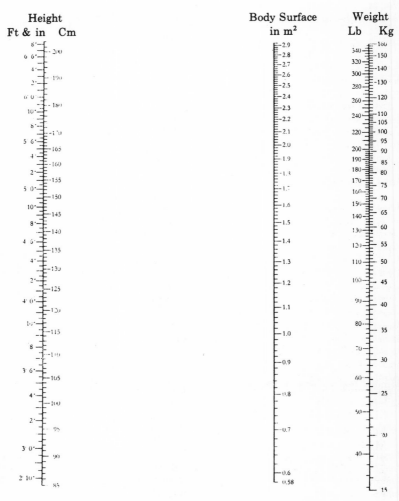

Nomogram of body weight, body height and body surface area.

Index

This index should not be used until you have read the book
1st bold figure(s) indicate chapter, the non-bold figure(s) refer to the paragraph.